The Heart Health Bible

ALSO BY JOHN M. KENNEDY:

The 15 Minute Heart Cure

The Heart
Health Bible

*The Five-Step Plan to Prevent
and Reverse Heart Disease*

John M. Kennedy, M.D.

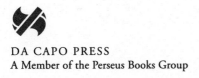

DA CAPO PRESS
A Member of the Perseus Books Group

Printed in the United States of America.

For information, address Da Capo Press, 44 Farnsworth Street, 3rd Floor, Boston, MA 02210.

Set in 12 point Adobe Garamond Pro by Marcovaldo Productions for the Perseus Books Group

Cataloging-in-Publication data for this book is available from the Library of Congress.
First Da Capo Press edition 2014
ISBN: 978-0-7382-1718-5 (paperback)
ISBN: 978-0-7382-1719-2 (eBook)

Published by Da Capo Press
A Member of the Perseus Books Group
www.dacapopress.com

Da Capo Press books are available at special discounts for bulk purchases in the U.S. by corporations, institutions, and other organizations. For more information, please contact the Special Markets Department at the Perseus Books Group, 2300 Chestnut Street, Suite 200, Philadelphia, PA, 19103, or call (800) 810-4145, ext. 5000, or e-mail special.markets@ perseusbooks.com.

10 9 8 7 6 5 4 3 2 1

To my beautiful family
Jayanna, Emily & Alexa

Prevention is better than cure.

—ERASMUS

CONTENTS

PART III   A Heart Healthy Future

The Heart Health Bible

Introduction

It was more than forty years ago on a beautiful sunny afternoon when I first sat down on a hand crafted wooden bench made by my Italian grandfather in St. Helena, California, the jewel of the famed Napa County wine country. Every Sunday without fail, over thirty aunts, uncles, cousins, nieces, and nephews would gather for a multi-course meal created by my grandparents.

I still recall the rays of sunlight skirting through the grapevines, which covered the wooden latticework that offered shade to a large outdoor dining table. The meal always started with an acknowledgment of family members, helping foster a collective sense of togetherness.

First course always was salad with sliced tomatoes, drenched with extra virgin olive oil, fresh rosemary, and garlic from my grandparents' garden and homemade wine vinegar. From there, we moved on to antipasto, pasta, and the main course, usually a delicious chicken or fish dish cooked over an outdoor grill. We followed up our meal with a twenty-minute walk and then returned home for a competitive game of bocce ball. Later on, we'd all share in an assortment of delicious homemade desserts, long goodbyes, and talk of next week's meal.

After twenty years as clinical cardiologist, I realize how prophetic my grandparents, great aunts, and uncles really were. All lived into their nineties, one even hit the 100 mark, and they say that diet and exercise were keys to their longevity and good health. I would argue that it was more. I believe their behavior and unwavering commitment to a heart-healthy lifestyle including stress reduction, healthy diet, and regular physical activity all contributed equally. Their sense of community, family, and enjoying the moment cannot be overlooked.

As cardiologists we're taught to follow evidence-based medicine where the medications, therapies, and surgical techniques we prescribe are determined and supported by scientific studies. We're well aware of the critical role behavior plays in achieving optimal heart health. A combination of healthy diet, stress reduction, and regular exercise can reduce the risk of heart attack and need for surgery. Adopting healthier lifestyle habits, which I'll discuss throughout the book, can help those diagnosed with atherosclerosis—the disease that causes heart attacks—slow and even reverse coronary heart disease. There's ample evidence human behavior is the most critical factor in reversing and preventing heart disease and achieving optimal heart health.

Personally, I've always wondered why heart disease remains the number one killer year after year, and I have always known that thousands of deaths could be prevented if only a simple template describing how to get it done were available. Imagine if the numbers are correct: that anywhere from 200,000–800,000 heart disease related deaths each year could be prevented through lifestyle changes alone. Achieving this goal may be easier said than done. A heart-healthy lifestyle requires dedication and commitment.

Throughout my training and my practice in clinical cardiology I have seen various diets and the latest exercise fads come and go. *The Heart Health Bible* separates itself from the clutter. Instead of emphasizing a new diet or trendy exercise, this book is about changing behavior using a simple, five-step template.

In addition, the book is filled with anecdotes and stories you may connect to, natural ways to protect and optimize your heart, and heart-healthy recipes created from foods shown to help your heart. This book is designed to be interactive, and encourages you to follow your H-E-A-R-T by tracking, logging and recording your results. The book is also filled with resources applicable to clinicians and patients alike.

HOW THIS BOOK WORKS

I believe that in order to adopt and maintain a heart-healthy lifestyle one needs a clear and simple template to follow, which is why I created H-E-A-R-T where each of the five letters represents an essential behavior and step designed to help protect and optimize your heart. Each chapter begins with a familiar story followed by discussion of one of the five steps.

Throughout the book you will learn that as we gain weight our blood pressure rises, we become less physically active, our waist size increases, and our blood sugar and cholesterol rises. To help remedy this internal cascade you will learn to:

Heal your blood pressure
Energize your heart
Act on fat
Reduce blood sugar
Tackle Triglycerides

As you read each chapter concentrate on each of the five steps discussed and learn how these actions and behaviors will help you achieve your ideal five numbers.

You will notice that there are both specifics and overlap for achieving all five and for achieving optimal heart health.

At the end of the chapter reflect on the topic and numbers discussed, then write down your number, and, based on recommendations, make a plan to achieve your ideal number.

For example:

At end of hypertension/"Your Blood Under Pressure" chapter, write your number down:

Yours	Ideal BP
152/90	<140/90

How to "H—Heal your blood pressure":

Watch a sunset today.

Watch your salt intake (< 1.5 gm/d).

Drink less alcohol or don't drink.

Walk for twenty minutes at lunch today.

Eat a banana and include tomatoes and broccoli in a salad.

Changing your mind and adopting these behaviors will lead to a literal everlasting change of H-E-A-R-T.

PART I

Welcome to the Five-Step Plan

CHAPTER 1

A Preventable Disease If You Follow Your H-E-A-R-T

Hippocrates, often described as the founder of modern medicine, held that good health was a natural state and disease an abnormality. Always, his work focused on assisting nature to help our bodies achieve this ideal. Hippocrates stressed the importance of disease prevention, and not simply the treatment or management of symptoms. Sounds great in theory but how does it work in practice? After all, we're a society that doesn't act until the wheels fall off the wagon. Nowhere does this sentiment ring truer than in the realm of heart disease. Today, the great irony of heart disease is that it's the most common, costly, and deadly of all health problems, but also the most preventable. Sadly, we're not taking enough steps in the prevention direction, opting instead for costly and invasive medical interventions and medications that alleviate symptoms but don't really address the underlying problem. But with heart disease still the leading cause of death and disability in America, and with 75 percent of our healthcare dollars spent on treating chronic conditions, we can't wait. We can't afford to ignore our H-E-A-R-T anymore.

Today, prevention is no longer a choice—it's a necessity. This chapter reminds you, by way of our friend Mr. Hippocrates, that our true *nature* is a healthy, pre-disease state. But I'd argue that an overreliance on technology to solve problems we can better fix ourselves has caused us to lose a vital connection to our own bodies. Simply, we've lost our way. When it comes to our health, we're reactive rather than proactive. This doesn't work. Anyone can give you a pill, put in a stent, and unclog your artery. But those things in and of themselves aren't going to make you better. Technology helps but prevention works better, and here is the best part. It's free. As you read this chapter, I encourage you to shed the old ideas and faulty thinking that have led to premature disability, compromised quality of life, out-of-control medical costs, and millions of needless deaths. In its place, consider a paradigm for lasting cardiovascular health: H-E-A-R-T.

MARJORIE'S STORY: FOLLOW YOUR HEART

Marjorie knew the score. Just a year earlier, her brother, a married father of three, successful software designer and accomplished amateur athlete, collapsed and died of a massive heart attack while out for an early morning jog. At forty-four, Marjorie's sister underwent coronary artery bypass surgery. Both of her parents succumbed to congestive heart failure. Children can learn a lot from their families, especially whether they're at risk for cardiovascular disease. Marjorie knew this. Her doctor had spoken to her about her tragic family legacy. But as an overworked executive vice president at a Fortune 500 pharmaceutical firm, most days she barely had time to eat, much less pay attention to her health.

Indeed, Marjorie didn't get to the top by accident. At thirty, she was head of marketing for a major pharmaceutical firm. Just five years later, Marjorie was named Vice President for Operations. Here she was: A top-level executive at a major company before the age of forty. Along the way, Marjorie also acquired a very healthy salary and bank account. Sadly, Marjorie's salary and bank account were about the only "healthy" things in her life.

In her quest to the reach the top, Marjorie had all but ignored her health. Most mornings, she'd leave home before dawn, pausing only long enough to grab a large cup of black coffee, which she filled with multiple packets of sugar. Often, she'd skip breakfast, or grab whatever she could find at the office (a glazed donut and handful of Peanut M & M's were two of her favorites). Her daily exercise regimen consisted of making every excuse imaginable to stay out of the gym and remain glued to her comfortable office chair. She'd let almost a year slip by without exercise, unless you count speed-dialing Chinese takeout as exercise. High stress and no downtime are often the price tag for a cushy office, stock options, and six-figure income.

For Marjorie, everything changed two years ago, just a few days shy of her fortieth birthday. She'd just returned from a whirlwind five-day business trip when it felt like "someone had dropped a heavy weight on my chest," she would later recall. Within three hours, Marjorie was in the emergency room where the attending physician diagnosed her as an "overworked and stressed out executive." She was sent home and advised to get some rest and take it easy. But this advice didn't sit right with Marjorie. Intuitively, she knew something was wrong. On the suggestion of her uncle, who'd undergone balloon angioplasty and had a stent placed into one of his two main coronary arteries, Marjorie scheduled an appointment with me, where we learned that she had elevated blood cholesterol. An ECG test revealed that her heart's electrical activity was out of kilter, as were the results of a nuclear stress test, which measures blood flow to the heart. I promptly ordered cardiac catheterization—a procedure that injects dye into the coronary arteries to check for blockages.

Turns out, Marjorie didn't have just one blockage. Two of three major arteries in her heart were almost completely occluded. Though she'd been asymptomatic prior to the emergency room visit, Marjorie would certainly have had a major coronary event within the next few months.

Though the procedure to clear Marjorie's blocked arteries was a success, it didn't have to be this way. The months of missed work, the antiplatelet therapy, beta blockers, ACE inhibitors, and nearly a year of intensive cardiac rehabilitation could all have been avoided. Marjorie learned her lesson but it came at a very high price. By taking action years earlier, and by paying attention to her family history she could have all but eliminated her risk factors for heart disease.

Reflecting on her experience, Marjorie told me, "I want to be here. I don't want to be a cautionary tale. I almost died because I didn't listen and ignored the warning signs. I now see the value of being proactive."

While I was heartened by Marjorie's sudden about-face, and I'm happy to report she's doing much better, to this day I'm still troubled that it had to come to this. Why did it take a near tragedy for Marjorie to turn things around? And for every Marjorie, there are thousands whose stories don't end so well. I still recall one of my first experiences as a cardiology fellow in the ER of a San Francisco Bay Area hospital. It was late, well past midnight when my beeper went off. A young man, just thirty-one, had been brought to the ER complaining of acute chest pain, abdominal discomfort, and shortness of breath. He was anxious, sweating bullets, and nauseous. In other words, he was having a heart attack. As he lay there in the stretcher, with me by his side and two medical residents and a nurse gathered around, our new patient went into sudden cardiac arrest. With a heart attack, a clogged artery is often the guilty party, reducing the amount of oxygen or blood flow and causing the heart muscle to die. During cardiac arrest, the heart's sophisticated electrical system goes haywire. Simply, the heart just stops beating. CPR and ultimately defibrillation are needed immediately to shock the heart back into rhythm. After a half an hour with no success, we were forced to stop our prolonged and concerted efforts at resuscitation.

As the only cardiology fellow on duty that night, it was my job to inform his next of kin. The hardest part of being a doctor is telling family and friends that a loved one has died. It comes with the territory but it never gets easier. By the time I walked from acute care to the emergency waiting room, several members of the young man's family had gathered. Before uttering a word, my facial expression signaled that I wouldn't be bringing good news on this night. I was tired, at the tail end of thirty-six-hour shift, and don't even remember what I said. How do you tell family members that a cherished husband, father, bother and son isn't coming home? The young man's wife, pregnant with their first child, informed me that her husband had been home all day preparing their baby's nursery. Already he'd painted the walls, assembled the crib, put up curtains, and even arranged a collection of stuffed animals next to the changing table—a room ready for a life he would never witness.

Patients die—it's a fact of life. But even twenty years ago, long before prevention had become all the rage in allopathic medicine, I knew it didn't have to be this way. When asked, "Why…why did this happen" by the patient's family members, in all likelihood I fumbled through an explanation. But in truth, I intuitively knew the answer. This patient's death—like so many others who succumb to heart disease—could have been avoided. When someone dies in an emergency room there's always a mountain of paperwork to fill out. Reviewing the patient's medical history the next day, I learned that he had a long family history of heart disease, which always increases the risk for relatives. Both his father and uncle had suffered heart attacks. His older sister was treated for unstable angina, a condition where the heart doesn't get enough blood flow or oxygen. And my patient, while clearly a loving and devoted father and husband did little to take care of himself. He'd given little thought to the family history of heart disease, as he was severely overweight, smoked on and off since high school, and got little physical exercise. He had hyperlipidemia, or elevated blood lipid levels, as well as elevated blood cholesterol (the two are closely related) and high blood pressure.

To this day, I still don't have a good explanation as to why a young man with everything in the world to live for ignored his health. When my patient's wife asked, "why," I knew that I couldn't provide her with a satisfactory answer. I wasn't satisfied with the answers I gave myself. However, from that moment forward I realized that it would become my life's mission to reduce the number of times I heard that question.

THE GREAT AMERICAN PARADOX

The great irony of the twenty-first-century heart disease epidemic is that we know more about the causes of cardiovascular disease than at any time in medical history. Twenty years ago, terms like "metabolic syndrome" didn't exist in the scientific literature. Atherosclerosis was treated with open heart surgery. It was thought that large plaques literally blocked blood vessels, shutting down blood flow and triggering heart disease. Our ignorance also extended to lifestyle choices. When I started my medical training in the late 1980s, physicians were loath to make the connection between high cholesterol and atherosclerosis. Package warning labels on cigarettes didn't even mention "heart disease" until 1981. There was no connection between depression and heart disease. We had no clue that heart disease risk increases dramatically for people who spend more than two hours a day sitting.

We're in the dark no longer. Cutting-edge research has given us greater insight into the factors that increase the risk of a cardiovascular disease. More than sixty years after the first famous Framingham

Heart Study—commissioned by the Federal government to find out what was killing scores of healthy men in their fifties and sixties—we've pretty much cornered the market on the risk factors for cardiovascular disease. Family history, obesity, smoking, high fat diet, high blood pressure, elevated blood sugar, stress, lack of physical activity, depression, and diabetes represent just a handful. Cardiologists have unprecedented access to imaging technology that actually peers into our artery walls looking for the build-up of cholesterol plaques that can lead to a heart attack. There are drugs that increase HDL (good) cholesterol and lower LDL (bad) levels in just weeks, halting the progression of atherosclerosis and reducing vascular inflammation. Using information collected from the Human Genome Project, scientists have identified a new allele that appears to play a significant role in controlling triglyceride levels in the blood. Today, we can treat mitral regurgitation (MR), blood leakage through the mitral valve into the heart chamber, without risky and invasive open heart surgery. We know that the mind and emotions are powerful predictors of cardiac events and coronary artery disease. These great discoveries and cutting-edge technologies are just the tip of the iceberg in our effort to treat the scourge of heart disease.

But important questions are being overlooked. Why are more than 50,000 mitral valve surgical procedures performed annually in the U.S.? Why are there more than 500,000 angioplasties?[1] Why hasn't three decades of low fat propaganda and a steady increase in the number of people taking cholesterol-lowering drugs significantly reduced the frequency of coronary bypass surgery? With all that's known about heart disease, why do Americans still have a coronary event every twenty-five seconds? Why is cardiovascular disease still the leading cause of death in the United States and a major cause of disability? And if heart disease can be prevented, why do an estimated sixty million people in the U.S. suffer from some form of cardiovascular illness?[2]

MEDICINE ISN'T ALWAYS THE ANSWER

As an interventional cardiologist, it would be foolish for me to dismiss the enormous contributions modern medicine has made in treating and even reversing heart disease. Angioplasty, as an example, can be a lifesaver for someone in the throes of a heart attack. But heart attack victims represent just a fraction of the millions who undergo these costly and risky procedures.

Millions of patients, in fact, have no obvious cardiac symptoms of any sort. And these procedures in otherwise healthy patients may not reduce the risk of heart attacks or sudden cardiac death. It's possible that an unnecessary procedure is performed on stable patients. The reasons vary, but in some patients even with severe blockages in the coronary arteries, surgery and angioplasty and stunting might not be needed.

In a controversial and widely disseminated study that shook the foundations of interventional cardiology, researchers concluded that surgical angioplasty and stent placement yields negligible additional benefit when used with a cocktail of generic drugs in patients suffering from chronic chest pain. The "Courage" trial, which tracked 2,287 patients for five years, found that trying drugs first, and adding stents only if chest pain persisted, didn't affect death rates and heart attacks. Though stent implants dropped off 13 percent in the month after the study's release in 2007, stenting rose again once the sensational headlines faded, and are now hovering around a million per year.[3]

Our overreliance on technology doesn't stop at surgery. I have a patient, a physician actually, who insisted I perform a cardiac CT angiography after he experienced unstable angina and became enamored with this latest machinery. CT angiography is a radiological test that combines the technology of a conventional CT scan with that of traditional angiography to create detailed images of the blood vessels in the body. These tests, which bill anywhere from $500 to

$1,500 and up, have never been proved in large medical studies to be more dependable or accurate than older or cheaper tests. They expose patients to large doses of radiation equivalent to several hundred X-rays, upping the risk for cancer. But we keep doing them, risk and cost notwithstanding.[4]

Widespread use of cardiac CT tomography, coupled with invasive surgical procedures, is part of a growing and alarming trend in interventional cardiology that makes use of technologies even without proof that they're appropriate or can help forecast the risk of a cardiac event. And even if a CT angiogram turns up a blockage, that doesn't mean that treatment is warranted. Sometimes a clot breaks up by itself and blood supply is restored to the heart. Or, a narrowed coronary artery may develop new blood vessels called *coronary collaterals* that connect the larger vessels in the heart and circumvent the blockage. One study found that patients with lots of these vessels have a 36 percent reduced risk of mortality, buttressing their importance as a therapeutic target.[5] And here's the most important fact: High technology across the board is no more protective than following a heart-healthy lifestyle. But we continue to make use of everything we can get our hands on because invasive cardiology is a big buck business. On the other hand, there's almost no financial incentive for doctors to promote a prevention-based model. Counseling patients about healthy food choices, exercise, and stress management makes sense but it's not reimbursable. Preventive measures work as well if not better than conventional modalities, but there's no incentive for doctors to recommend them.

If the numbers are any indication, the "pound wise–penny foolish" approach—spending money on things we don't need—to treating heart disease doesn't work in the long run. In 2013 alone, it's estimated that cardiovascular disease will cost more than $450 billion in health care, medications, and lost productivity. That price tag is expected to triple by 2030, from $273 billion to $818 billion, a figure that doesn't even account for another $276 billion in lost productivity.[6] Perhaps if we redirected some of the cash spent on intervention to prevention, we'd have a much healthier—not to mention wealthier—population.

THE PROBLEM WITH THE PREVENTION MESSAGE

"An apple a day keeps the doctor away." We've been told for years that an ounce of prevention is the best medicine, especially when it comes to chronic problems like heart disease. The key to a good prevention strategy consists of minimizing and controlling the risk factors that contribute to disease. The general consensus in the field is that all modifiable risk factors for cardiovascular disease—those that don't include age, gender, and family history in other words—can be controlled with lifestyle modifications such as regular exercise, stress reduction, and a healthy diet.

But with all the good news about prevention, there's still a 5000-pound elephant in the room that no one wants to talk about. The emergence of a prevention-based model hasn't really curtailed the heart disease epidemic. All of our efforts to decrease smoking, reduce stress, promote a healthy diet, and highlight the benefits of regular physical activity haven't impacted the problem. Indeed, after a twenty-year decline in the rate of coronary artery disease, things might be trending in the opposite direction, as both heart disease and heart disease risk factors are again on the increase.[7,8]

Why isn't the message getting through? There's an interesting parallel between heart disease prevention and weight loss. Dieting is a $75 billion business in the U.S. At any time, a third of all Americans are on a diet. Yet, almost 69 percent of the U.S. population is still overweight or obese.[9] And here's a fact that no one wants to talk about: within months or years, the entire effort comes undone, and the average dieter has packed on the pounds again with interest. Indeed, two-thirds of dieters gain back the weight in a year and 97 percent gain it back within five years.[10] When it comes to weight control, the message isn't getting through. Though it's easy to point the finger at dieters for failing, perhaps it's the message that needs work.

Integrative cardiology is a big buzz phrase in field of heart disease prevention. It's a melding of the very best offerings from complimentary and conventional medicine. The effectiveness and importance of natural alternatives such as nutritional medicine, exercise, and stress reduction are emphasized. In other words, they talk about what we *should* do. We know what we should do. But there isn't a prevention model that considers what people really do. Indeed, behavioral change is the most daunting task facing anyone working in the field of chronic disease prevention. Today, we treat diabetes with genetically engineered synthetic insulin and even insulin analogues. Yet, diabetes is still skyrocketing. Why? Because diabetes is a complex behavioral disorder that requires people to make changes. Medicine doesn't make people change. I can tell you to exercise regularly, toss out the cigarettes, eat better, and reduce stress. But that knowledge goes nowhere if it's never implemented. And you won't implement anything without a change in mindset.

There are literally hundreds of programs for preventing and reversing heart disease. I can't think of a major medical center in this country that doesn't have a preventive cardiology program. But along the way, the notion of what prevention means—and what it's intended to prevent—has diffused. There's no coherent, unifying view of what's needed. We know that diet is critical. Weight, in fact, is the most modifiable risk factor for cardiovascular disease.

A well-known cardiologist posed the following question on his popular blog: "Why is there a reticence to provide the public with [dietary] guidelines that will spare them [heart disease] or its progression?" I'll tell you *why* there's reticence. Because the guidelines suggested by my otherwise well-intentioned colleague, which feature a diet consisting exclusively of whole grains, vegetables, fruits, and legumes, are impossible for the majority of people to adhere to.

There's nothing wrong with a plant-based diet. Nor would I challenge the efficacy of a vegetarian diet in reducing and preventing heart disease. But try getting compliance with a diet that doesn't include butter, eggs, cream, cheese, oils, ice cream, nuts, fish, poultry, and meat. As the National Research Council concluded, a dietary fat recommendation lower than 30 percent is too difficult for those looking to lose a lot of weight. For the majority of heart patients, the clarion call to "health" is secondary to the call of the foods they cherish. If the opposite were true, millions of people in this country might not have heart disease in the first place!

Extreme low fat diets may be of some scientific value, but they don't consider the full range of human experience. Eating is a pleasurable event for most people. Taste and texture arouse our taste buds, stimulating our brain's intricate reward system. Normally enjoyable activities like eating don't lend themselves to moderation but to excess. We can tell the public what we believe is best for their health, and even provide evidence to support our position. But if no one complies then there's no positive impact on health. It's as if the diet never existed.

TAKING THE PULSE OF PREVENTION

In medical school, one of the first things I learned is how to take a person's vital signs. Temperature, pulse, breathing and blood pressure—taken together, these four signs are the greatest indicator of a person's wellbeing. Though I didn't give it much thought at the time, it now seems appropriate that one of the first things l learned to do was to take a patient's pulse, a recording of the arteries expanding and recoiling during the systolic and diastolic phase of each cardiac cycle. In the nascent stage of human development, just three weeks after the sperm meets the egg, a process known as organogenesis takes place. Organogenesis means "that with which one works," and it signals the beginning of the embryonic phase when the three primary germ cell layers in the human embryo change and grow into internal organs. The circulatory system, and its companion organ—the heart—emerge during this third week. At that moment, the heart consists of little more than two tiny channels called heart tubes. Yet, these tubes are already hard at work. Stimulated by electrical impulses, they're beating and pumping blood, long before chambers and arteries form. This amazing clump of tissue keeps beating until you take your last breath.

Even when fully grown, the human heart is no bigger than the size of your fist. Yet, it's an extraordinary biological phenomenon. At the most basic level, the heart is a pump composed of muscle. It beats approximately 72 times per minute, 100,000 times a day, and 2.5 to 3 billion times in an average lifetime. The heart pumps blood, carrying the material needed to help our bodies' function and remove waste products we don't need.

For all our heart does, we spend most of our lives ignoring it. Most people, even those with heart disease, don't notice their heart until they have a cardiac event. But we need to recognize our heart as the most important organ. To paraphrase a line from the Bible, "Above all else, guard your heart, for it affects everything you do."

It's been said that we live in the age of experience. The advent of the microchip has ushered in a new era, defined by personal computing, 24–7 Internet access, digital media, and device proliferation. As we rush through life at break neck speed, this new technology helps us connect to the world and to each other whether we're sharing photos of our children, or Skyping with colleagues on the other side of the globe. Action and reaction, we're constantly touching and feeling the outside world through this remarkable technology.

Ironically, we never acknowledge what makes these actions possible. It is, in fact, our beating heart that guides our thoughts and actions throughout these frenzied days. We must acknowledge, touch, and feel our hearts with the same unbridled enthusiasm we have for our smart phones.

CHANGING MINDS: FEELING THE PULSE

Among modern medicine's many contributions, there's a general consensus that the germ theory of disease has done more for the welfare of the world's people than any other discovery. The work of pioneering microbiologists like Ignaz Semmelweis, Louis Pasteur, and Joseph Lister helped to explain why millions of soldiers during combat were more likely to die from staph infections than bullets. Germ theory opened whole new fields of research, and still guide health care practices to the present day. That's the power of an accurate paradigm. It explains, and then it guides.

"Paradigm" and "paradigm shift" are not every day words but they're powerful concepts. Paradigm comes from the Greek *paradeigma*, once exclusively a scientific term but it's now taken to mean a perception, assumption, theory, frame of reference, or lens through which one views the world. Really, it's like getting a set of directions to a friend's house. If inaccurate, you'll get lost no matter how much effort you apply to finding your way. Diligence, outlook, and attitude matter only if the directions are spot on.

Albert Einstein once said, "The significant problems we face cannot be solved at the same level of thinking we were at when we created them." Einstein's profundity underscores a major point I'll make throughout this book: If we want to change the course of heart disease, we must change our thinking. The current approach to heart disease prevention is crying out for a paradigm shift. The message is being preached but it doesn't have enough adherents.

That's where H-E-A-R-T comes into play. H-E-A-R-T is an easy-to-follow, lifestyle enrichment method designed to eliminate disease risk factors through reducing blood cholesterol, triglycerides, and blood sugar levels by eliminating excess weight, lowering high blood pressure, adopting daily exercise, and improving dietary choices that can prevent and reverse disease. It's my firm belief that H-E-A-R-T will become a daily reminder and template for thousands looking to decrease the risk of cardiac events while optimizing their heart health.

Accordingly, this book calls on you to acknowledge your H-E-A-R-T in each and everything you do, whether you're eating, exercising, or dealing with life's unexpected challenges and misfortunes. Once you acknowledge your H-E-A-R-T you can take steps to guard it.

H-E-A-R-T marks a shift away from invasive, costly, and risky interventions to noninvasive approaches aimed at early detection and prevention. By and large, conventional medicine has dropped the ball and taken people down the wrong path. To borrow a well-worn idiom, it's as if we're forever closing the barn door after the horses have already escaped. For a majority of people, heart disease is a symptom, not the cause of their problems. We should be teaching people ways to avoid heart disease before it ever starts, or at least to halt and reverse its course. As I tell patients, the power to stay healthy is in your hands. But the key lies in following your H-E-A R-T.

Given the high cost of treating acute and chronic disease, prevention offers the potential of improving health and cutting costs. What we're currently spending on treating cardiovascular disease isn't sustainable. However, we can afford to prevent it. Indeed, we can't afford not to. That's why we need our H-E-A-R-T.

Prevention pays for itself, both monetarily and also by lengthening and improving the quality of life. More important, prevention doesn't just affect us today. It will have a positive impact on generations to come. Indeed, healing the unhealthy pulse of our nation begins by learning to acknowledge, feel and protect our own H-E-A-R-T.

H-E-A-R-T is a new way of life—a heart-healthy way of life. Though it's easy to follow, H-E-A-R-T is a way of life that some will find challenging. But the challenge is one that should be welcomed and embraced. In fact, if your goals include living a long and healthy life, this challenge must be welcomed. As long as you're alive, it's never too late to follow your H-E-A-R-T.

CHAPTER 2

Five Steps That Will Save Your Life

This chapter turns a critical eye to the current state of heart health in the United States. Despite recent advances in heart disease treatment, and an untold number of bells, whistles, and toys that help people with a wide range of conditions, odds are that most of us will die from some form of cardiovascular disease. Indeed, cardiovascular disease claims more lives than the next four leading causes—cancer, accidents, respiratory illness, and diabetes—combined. We know this, yet millions continue with lifestyle choices that damage their heart and increase their risk cardiovascular disease. This chapter introduces readers to my perspective on heart disease and why the zeitgeist needs to change. Of course, optimal heart health will remain out of reach if we simply follow the old formula of treating symptoms instead of addressing the underlying causes. Therefore, we need H-E-A-R-T, my easy-to-follow, heart-healthy lifestyle method—a daily reminder and template designed to protect and optimize our most precious and vital organ. Throughout *The Heart Health Bible*, I refer to **H-E-A-R-T**, an acronym that will help you acknowledge, understand and take five action steps:

1. **H**eal high blood pressure
2. **E**nergize for a strong, healthy heart
3. **A**ct against fat
4. **R**educe blood sugar
5. **T**ackle triglycerides

These five steps are aimed at decreasing the risk of a cardiovascular event and enhancing your heart health. In this chapter, I explain each of the steps, what they mean, and how they act together and independently to decrease the risk of a cardiovascular event.

KARA'S STORY: FALLING ON DEAF EARS

"Honestly doctor, I don't have time for this today."

It's a warm, early June morning and Kara, a junior partner in a firm specializing in patent law, is sitting in her internist's office, just a stone's throw from downtown Los Angeles, reacting to the results of her annual physical. The internist had just delivered a dose of news Kara was in no mood to hear. "Your LDL cholesterol and your triglycerides are through the roof, you're carrying excess fat around your middle, and you've got hypertension," she told Kara, who was now busily texting her assistant and only half listening to her well-intentioned doctor. "O.K. I heard you. So now what?" replied Kara, barely pausing long enough to make eye contact. "Well, this is a serious issue, Kara. But I do have some suggestions for lowering your cholesterol and triglycerides and getting blood pressure under control," said the doctor. "Can you fill me in quickly, doc? I have a partner's-only meeting in half hour," Kara replied impatiently. Kara's doctor, a polite, genial woman who'd been at this a long time, seemed taken aback by her patient's curt response, particularly given the severity of the diagnosis. "This is a serious issue, Kara. We're talking about your life." Kara seemed impervious to her doctor's comments and far more concerned with the flurry of text messages coming through her iPhone. Nevertheless, the doctor pressed ahead, as any good physician would. "Well, I'm going to suggest some things, lifestyle modifications for the most part," she said, pointing out that if Kara just added a bit more fruit and vegetables to her diet, cut out some of the crap—no more donuts and caramel lattes for breakfast—and committed to some form of moderate exercise, in one to two weeks she'd start to see those numbers drop.

"Look, I'm swamped," Kara told her doctor. "Most days, I scarcely have a moment to brush my teeth. Now you're telling me to add exercise and spend time preparing healthy foods. I can't do it. I don't have the time. Can't you just give me some medication? My dad was taking something…statins, maybe something else I think. I could do that."

In fact, Kara's dad, who also suffered from high cholesterol and hypertension, was taking Crestor, a statin, and a beta-blocker combined with a thiazide diuretic to open his blood vessels to lower the workload on his heart. But less than a year after starting this medication regimen, Kara's dad suffered a massive heart attack, which left him permanently disabled. How is this possible? After all, he was taking the most powerful hypertension and cholesterol-lowering medications on the market. How is it that drugs that do all the right things—lower bad cholesterol, raise good cholesterol, and lower blood pressure—could raise the risk of heart disease and even death?

There was only one small problem—in taking these drugs, Kara's dad never had to address the underlying cause of his high cholesterol and hypertension: His lifestyle, behavior, and attitude. We're back to the proverbial 5,000 pound elephant. These drugs didn't treat the underlying cause of his cardiovascular problems. To my knowledge, we have yet to develop a drug that counteracts the effects of overeating high calorie, processed foods, marital discord, and persistent nihilism. Drugs have limited value in helping people with chronic health conditions like hypertension and high cholesterol because as we'll see again and again in this book, pills don't make people. From cancer to diabetes, all chronic health conditions share a strong, underlying behavioral component that can't be addressed with a pill, injection, dietary supplement, or surgical procedure. In fact, they often exacerbate the problem because they give people an easy out. By and large, the cause(s) of chronic diseases are rooted in what we eat, how much we move/exercise, how we cope with stress, the quality of our relationships, and our ambient environment.

At best, these new super drugs will help lower cholesterol numbers and reign in hypertension without too many debilitating side effects. But no drug, no matter how effective, addresses the fact that cardiovascular disease isn't a simple Crestor or beta-blocker problem. Thus, it can't simply be "fixed" with a prescription medication, surgical intervention, or dietary supplement. Cardiovascular illness is the result of an intricate mosaic fueled by diet, physical activity, stress, and other lifestyle factors such as smoking, social connections, and, increasingly, even environmental hazards/toxins. Pills don't address these critical variables. Pills don't arrest problems that push our biology steadily along the path of heart disease. The idea of using statins or a combination of beta blocker and thiazide diuretics to fix heart disease is a classic example of a problem besetting medical science: Cartesian, reductionist thinking. High cholesterol and hypertension aren't Kara's problems—just as they weren't problems for her father per se. They're symptoms. The problem for Kara and her dad—decent, well-intentioned, and hardworking people—is their thinking. It's flawed thinking that affects behavior and pushes millions down the road to heart disease.

Kara and her father, both of whom became my patients, are cautionary tales of a phenomenon I see sweeping allopathic medicine: palliation of symptoms without any thought to dealing with the cause of the disease. Kara's internist, at least, was on the right track. She knew that her patient's abnormally high cholesterol and hypertension were just a downstream problem resulting from poor lifestyle choices and an inherited tendency for cynicism rather than an underlying medical condition or long family history of heart disease. Everything Kara did to herself she could undo. Not through taking a statin, CETP inhibitor, or Bystolic. These medications wouldn't reverse changes in her biology—any more than they did for her father—which at the time of her visit with her internist could safely be labeled as "diabesity," Dr. Mark Hyman's term to describe a continuum of abnormal biology that ranges from mild insulin resistance to full-blown diabetes. According to Dr. Hyman, diabesity affects 50 percent of adult Americans and is the leading cause of most chronic disease. More important, they weren't going to change her thinking and subsequent behavior, which was at the root of her cardiovascular problems.[1]

Drugs wouldn't reverse the changes brought on by a high sugar and refined flour, low fiber, processed diet, physical inactivity, excessive stress, sleep deprivation, or the harmful effects of environmental pollution. In fact, once Kara started taking Crestor, her total cholesterol was 173, and her LDL was 99. (An LDL of less than 100 milligrams per deciliter (mg/dL) is optimal.) But the good news ended there. Kara's triglycerides were 179 (normal is less than 100), and her HDL or "good" cholesterol was 37 (normal is greater than 50). High triglyceride levels may lead to heart disease, especially in people with low levels of "good" cholesterol and high levels of "bad" cholesterol, like Kara.

Kara was destined for a lifetime of serious, life threatening health problems. But unless she was willing to change her thinking, the effectiveness of any medical intervention would prove short-lived. As Kara and I spoke about her health problems, I painted a picture of what she could be in store for if changes weren't made and fast. "Look Kara, numbers don't lie. You've got four major risk factors for heart disease. If things continue, you could end up in the same boat as your dad."

Kara seemed puzzled. "Dr. Kennedy, you tell me I have all of these risk factors for heart disease. But I have to tell you I feel fine." "You may feel fine now and may never have experienced any symptoms. But heart disease is a 'silent killer' because it seldom reveals any symptoms," I countered. I shared with Kara that 50 percent of women and two-thirds of men their first time ever presenting with heart disease is either a heart attack or sudden cardiac death. Kara weighed my words carefully but still didn't seem convinced. Eventually, I sent Kara on her way with a prescription for a statin, antihypertensive, and a list of foods and exercises that could help reduce her abnormally high numbers.

I felt a sad after Kara left my office. Yet, I shouldn't have been entirely surprised since patients such as Kara are more the rule than the exception. For every patient who follows H-E-A-R-T or any other prevention model, there are dozens more who look for band aid solutions, resist treatment, or are just truculent, insisting they know better or don't have the time or interest in making the effort needed to change. Kara's story reminded me of how many at risk patients feel "paradoxically protected," as I told a colleague recently. "Dr. Kennedy, I can't feel my high blood pressure, high cholesterol, or high blood glucose. I don't notice any symptoms. I don't feel sick. What's the problem?"

For Kara, and millions more naysayers like her who are reluctant or unwilling to take action, and don't see the value in a preemptive "first strike," I've found that a "seeing is believing" approach works. Many a patients are literally "scared straight" after I share a photo of the inner lining of a blocked blood vessel. And a recent study showed that asymptomatic patients with high cholesterol were more likely to take cholesterol-lowering medication when they had cardiac CT-scans confirming the presence of disease.[2]

But graphic displays notwithstanding, just as often it seems the message doesn't get through. As a cardiologist, it's frustrating to hear patients say, "they don't feel anything" despite having high blood pressure, high cholesterol, high blood sugar, or any other number of risk factors. It's amazing that even a graphic photo of a plaque-strewn artery underway isn't motivation enough for them to change. If they don't feel anything, they don't see the need to rock the boat.

But rocking the boat is exactly what's needed. Across the globe, heart disease is reaching epidemic proportions. We've all heard the numbers and they're frightening.

Heart disease is the leading cause of death for both men and women in the United States, claiming approximately 1 million lives annually. By 2020, heart disease will be the leading cause of death throughout the world.

This year more than 920,000 Americans will have a heart attack; nearly half of them will occur without prior symptoms or warning signs. 250,000 Americans die annually of Sudden Cardiac Death—680 every day of the year.

Every 33 seconds someone in the United States dies from cardiovascular disease which is roughly the equivalent of a September 11th-like tragedy repeating itself every 24 hours, 365 days a year.

More people die of heart disease than of AIDS and all cancers combined.

An estimated 80 million Americans have one or more types of heart disease.

Currently about 7.9 million Americans are alive who have had a heart attack.

In 2008, the total cost of cardiovascular disease (coronary heart disease, hypertensive disease, heart failure, and stroke) in the U.S. was estimated at $448.5 billion. (This includes direct costs such as costs of doctors, hospital services, medications, etc., and indirect costs such as lost productivity.) In comparison, the estimated economic cost of cancer in 2007 was $219 billion.[3]

WHAT THE HECK IS GOING ON WITH HEART DISEASE?

Of course, these numbers represent just the tip of the heart disease iceberg. But just how did we get there? Why in an era when we've created technology that's pushed us to the forefront in the diagnosis, treatment, and management of cardiovascular illness, are more and more people continuing to fall victim to heart disease?

On the surface, heart disease is a strange illness, since the vast majority of us are born with ideal cardiovascular health. In fact, heart disease is largely an acquired illness. Certainly, the modern lifestyle is a factor. As an important article in the prestigious *American Journal of Lifestyle Medicine* points out, "In many ways, coronary heart disease represents the quintessential lifestyle disease of developed countries. Six of the major risk factors for developing CHD involve lifestyle practices, including the decision of whether or not to smoke, the control of blood pressure and lipids, diabetes, level of physical activity, and obesity."[4] Indeed, our sedentary lifestyle, smoking, stress, and consumption of large portions of unhealthy, high calorie foods are key reasons for our continuing struggle with heart disease.

And let's be even more blunt: We're fat. Today, almost 70 percent of adult Americans are overweight or obese. This number is expected to rise anywhere from 60 to 80 percent by 2030 if trends continue (and I've seen nothing to indicate they won't).[5] And the worst part is that we carry a majority of this excess weight around our middle. Beyond being unsightly and keeping us out of our skinny jeans, this type of deep or "visceral" fat lies inside our abdomen, surrounding our internal organs. Regardless of your overall weight, the proverbial potbelly increases your risk of cardiovascular disease and diabetes. Obesity has now supplanted cigarette smoking as a major risk factor for premature death.

Not only are we fat, but also we're lazy. Particularly in the last twenty years, we've become wedded to and overly reliant upon modern conveniences that encourage a sedentary lifestyle, and have no doubt played a major role in this country's overweight and obesity epidemic. Our move from the field to the computer screen has wreaked havoc on our heart, which needs work to keep going, just like any other muscle. Certainly, there are millions of stressed-out, overworked adults and kids who don't have, or simply don't make time for exercise. But in another of the modern society's great ironies, more and more people are exercising but the national obesity rate keeps rising. During the last decade, Americans have gotten more active while also getting fatter in two-thirds of the nation's counties. Take my home state of California as an example. Across the state, the percentage of women who get sufficient weekly exercise rose over the past ten years from 50.7 percent to 59.2 percent. For men, the positive change was from 59.4 percent to 61.3 percent. Yet, at the same time, obesity rates rose in every California county![6,7]

Kids are suffering equally. Physical education programs are no longer mandatory and hundreds of school districts across the country have cut back on gym classes. Thus, kids today find themselves in similarly dire straits. It's estimated that only half of America's youth meet the current evidence-based guideline of the U.S. Health and Human Services Department of at least sixty minutes of vigorous or moderate-intensity physical activity daily. In my opinion, that number is much lower. It's unrealistic to think that given the current budget crunch at schools across the country that states will look at the research that shows the consequences of limited physical activity and immediately expand physical education programs. It is a tragic fact, and one that I see every day in my practice, that this generation of obese children may have shorter life expectancies than their parents. This puts heart disease in the category of modern day plague.

We eat too much, of course. Across the board, food portion sizes have grown, doubling in the last twenty years alone, to match our burgeoning waistlines. But we also eat really bad food. Though other nations are slowly making headway, we still hold the dubious distinction as the world's greatest consumers of unhealthy fats, refined carbohydrates, and excess calories. The average American diet consists of any number of well-known heart disease contributors including laboratory-produced trans fats, refined carbohydrates and sweets. Unstable blood sugar and elevated insulin levels, which propagate inflammation via a cascade of biochemical and hormonal changes, are the end game of these ill-conceived food choices. This sort of eating behavior can, and most often does lead to high LDL (bad) cholesterol and triglyceride levels. Adding to our ever-expanding stomachs and high blood pressure—triggered in part by insulin resistance—is the much dreaded metabolic syndrome or syndrome X, which I'll discuss at length in the next chapter. Metabolic syndrome didn't even exist when I was a kid.

Funny thing is that there shouldn't be anything wrong with *processed food*. Contrary to what many have come to believe, not all processed foods are "Franken foods," as the acclaimed journalist Michael Specter observed in his bestselling book, *Denialism: How Irrational Thinking Hinders Scientific Progress, Harms the Planet, and Threatens Our Lives.* "Moving molecules around in a specific, rather than a haphazard way isn't trespassing on nature's ground," observed Mr. Specter in a recent Ted talk. Three quarters of U.S. farmed corn and nearly 80 percent of soy comes from genetically modified seeds. Indeed, we monkey around with everything we eat—even the healthiest vegetables. We've manufactured a majority of the foods we eat over the last 10,000 years, Specter points out. The technology now exists to put Vitamin A into rice, which can help millions of people. That's a great development. In the next fifty years, we're going to have to grow 70 percent more food. That's possible only with fairly recent innovations in crop growing and biotechnology. We have no choice but to tinker with Mother Nature.[8,9]

Yet, so many of our health woes, including diabetes, obesity, and heart disease, which affect 50 percent of all Americans, and contribute to seven of every ten deaths in the U.S., didn't come out of the blue. Though such trends can't be easily explained by any one factor, the calorie-dense, additive-laden American diet hasn't helped matters.

HEART DISEASE: ONE MORE VIEW

Beyond the obvious lifestyle variables, there's another, less discussed component contributing to the rise in heart disease. Despite all the talk about the value of being proactive, as a society we're the opposite, especially when it comes to our health. It is one of least recognized truths of human behavior: We don't react until the wheels fall off the wagon. A bridge collapses. Someone shoots up an elementary school. A hurricane ravages the East Coast of the U.S. A terrorist bomb goes off during a marathon. Some married politician gets caught with his an underage intern. It seems that every new disaster brings about a call for change. This isn't a bad thing. After all, at least it shows that we care.

The problem is that a few days later we're off focusing on something else. Even the most odious tragedies seem to fade quickly from our collective consciousness. In part, we do this out of necessity. Our minds are designed to move us away from the memory of unpleasant experiences. It's a built-in survival mechanism. But our short attention spans, so critical for our survival on the one hand, have played havoc with our health on the other. We ignore our health and we react only after something horrible takes place. We get sick, and *then* we get scared. We vow to do anything to get better. We visit the doctor, who palliates our symptoms with a pill or procedure, without every really getting to the cause of the illness. The result: As soon as we start feeling better, we return to the old habits, and wait for the next crisis to consume our attention.

When it comes to our health, we only focus on issues when they blow up in our face. Even the "threat" of impending disaster, isn't enough for many of us to change, as we saw with my patient Kara. When it comes to our health, we spend a great deal of time reacting to, situations and circumstances, rather than creating and shaping them.

Why don't we make better decisions? Why do we wait for reality to beat us over the head? Despite, the obvious toll on our physical, psychological and financial well-being, why do we follow the destructive and demoralizing pattern of reacting, coping, and then returning to the way of the living that got us into trouble in the first place? Albert Einstein defined insanity as doing the same thing again and again and expecting a different result. I think the old man knew a good deal more about the human condition than most psychiatrists.

Part of the fault lies with modern medicine. We've provided a safety net for patients. They know there's an easy way out. We'll clean out their blocked arteries or give them a pill to control their hypertension, without every really insisting they tangibly change the behaviors and choices that got them into trouble in the first place. Technology and the willingness of many doctors to alleviate symptoms have contributed to the influx of reactive decision making. Why? It goes back to the point I made in the first chapter. Technology doesn't make people change. No doctor, no matter how skilled, can ever truly help a patient who's unwilling think differently about his or her health.

THE PATH TO LASTING CHANGE

In nature, there are basically two kinds of change: evolutionary and disruptive. *Evolutionary change* is what its name implies. It's somewhat gentler, less destructive, and happens organically. But it takes a very long time. On the other hand, disruptive change is fast, and sometimes necessary—but it can be extremely destructive, as we learned from the lessons of Hurricane Sandy. Human beings are clever a bunch, though. We've figured out how to speed up evolutionary change (genetic engineering and stem cell therapy) and how to manage and contain disruptive change (controlled forest fires and population control of indigenous animal species).

Which brings me to the idea of changing the health culture in the country. Taking a page from life, we change evolutionarily or disruptively. But since we're facing a heart health crisis in this country, and can't wait a couple hundred years to fix the problem, evolutionary change isn't enough. We need to speed things up, but in a way that produces real, lasting change.

Picture this scenario: You visit the dentist, who tells you the pain in your jaw is from a two cavities. You take care of it. Problem solved. Or is it? What are you going to do once the problem has been fixed? Are you going to still eat sweets? Are you going to forget to floss before brushing? Once the pain has passed what are you going to do to remind yourself of the thinking and behavior that got you in trouble?

Whenever a task seems overwhelming, it's always best to start small and slow. Instead of a paradigm shift, think of a few little things you can do right now. If you're afternoon snack consists of potato chips and a bottle of Coke, one day a week try replacing them with an apple and bottle of water. Going *cold turkey* is ideal but unrealistic for a majority of people. It's also the surest way to feel deprived, a key reason why dieters fail to keep weight off. Changing to a completely different way of doing business overnight is overwhelming. Old habits really do die hard. That's why I tell patients to choose the behaviors that will have the greatest impact on their cardiovascular health.

Too often, I see patients opt for the disruptive change, which might seem ideal particularly in the case of a noxious and dangerous habit like smoking, but it's highly unrealistic and untenable. This is why smokers looking to kick the habit take Chantix, or stick a Nicoderm patch on their arms. This is called agonist therapy—usually long-acting medications that stimulate the same brain receptors as the addictive drug. But changing deeply rooted behaviors—better known as habits—requires a change in thinking. This is the most vexing problem for those of us working in the field of preventive cardiology. How do we bring about real, lasting change that will positively impact our cardiovascular health?

In previous generations, the doctor/patient relationship was a structured, organized hierarchy. Sick? You visit the doctor. This was your sole source of health information. He'd give you a pill and you'd go home. You acted and interacted in prescribed ways. There was no Internet; 24–7 access to health information didn't exist. No one talked about the value of prevention.

Our health and our relationship to it have changed dramatically over the last few years. Today, anyone can look up information that was once under the purview of healthcare professionals. With a mouse click, my eight-year-old can access the latest information from medical journals (not that she'd understand anything she'd read in them). Our hopes, dreams, fears, and motivations have an enormous impact on our health. As physicians, we need to help people make sense of it all. We need to change with the times. We can't ignore this new health culture, which have been both a burden and a blessing.

But what is the path to lasting change? How do we prevent problems from surfacing in the first place?

How do we establish positive patterns of thinking and behavior, and then create the tools needed to promote and reinforce a lifetime of optimal cardiovascular health?

Fortunately, this isn't as hard as you may think. For years, I've been telling patients that even the most ingrained habits and intractable behaviors can be changed, but only if you know what's needed to move forward

After seeing more than 5,000 patients over twenty years as a practicing cardiologist, I firmly believe that people will change their thinking and subsequent behavior if they see that change as *Easy, Rewarding, and Normal.*

EASY: If I'm going to ask you to think or behave differently then I have to condition you to believe that *you already have at your disposal the necessary skills and tools, and there's nothing blocking your path to optimal cardiovascular health.* Change is hard for everyone, particularly if they don't have the right strategies and skills, or they encounter an obstacle along the way that seems insurmountable.

REWARDING: For a behavior to be rewarding, you have to believe that *you're going to get immediate, lasting results that will positively impact your health.* This is how behavior connects to thinking: I have to show you how a new way of thinking will lead to a change in behavior. For example, if I tell you to lower your blood pressure, I won't get very far unless I convince you of the importance of doing so, and then implement a positive behavior or set of behaviors that supports that goal. If I show you that practicing my *Breathe Technique can help your blood pressure in just ten-to-fifteen minutes a day, and it produces an immediate, tangible and positive result on your health then you might be more inclined to adopt this as part of your regular routine.*

NORMAL: This is the icing on the cake. In order to change your behavior, you're going to have to feel that anything I tell you is part of a normal heart-healthy lifestyle. First, you're going to have shed a lot of your old, faulty thinking. You're going to have to let go of the idea that every problem can be easily fixed with medical intervention. You're going have to realize that portion sizes that scarcely fit on your dinner plate are normal. You're going to have to realize that you do have time to exercise. I want you to behave differently. I want you to believe that our natural state is one that doesn't include high blood pressure, elevated LDL cholesterol, high blood sugar, a spare tire around the waist, 3000-calories a day of food, and surgical attachment to a remote control, so I have to give you evidence that what you're doing isn't working and that there is a better way.

Together, we need to figure out what needs to change, and how to make our shared goal of optimal heart health easier, more rewarding and more natural than the old way of doing business. It's not that we need to avoid problems. Stress, as an example, is unavoidable part of daily life. Stress itself isn't the issue. How we deal with stress is the issue.

FOLLOW YOUR H-E-A-R-T

After more than twenty years of practicing medicine, and witnessing firsthand the damage the modern, supercharged lifestyle has on our hearts, I find myself asking the same questions again and again: How can I change the conversation? Is there something I can do for today that would tangibly lessen my patients' risk of experiencing a cardiovascular event? From controlling high blood pressure and lowering bad cholesterol to managing the effects of stress and getting enough sleep, how do I get you to start thinking everyday about your heart?

For years, I've fantasized about having one reference that can help anyone—irrespective of her gender, race, age, and state of health—achieve optimal heart health without costly and invasive medical intervention. If there were such a tool, would heart attacks rapidly decline? Could it help make heart disease a thing of the past? Would it lead to a paradigm shift in the maladaptive thinking and unhealthy behaviors and habits that lead millions down the road to poor cardiovascular health? What if everyone knew about normal blood pressure, a proper exercise regimen, optimal waist size, and body mass index, how to lower and control their blood sugar, and the X's and O's of managing cholesterol?

At first glance, optimal heart health seems like a daunting task. It's no accident that heart disease is the leading cause of death for both men and women. The great news is that in most cases, all optimal heart health can be achieved without a doctor's prescription. But don't expect a quick fix. When it comes to reversing and ultimately preventing heart disease, there is no such thing as lightning in a bottle. Achieving and more importantly maintaining a healthy heart requires commitment and dedication. To smooth the road ahead, I've created a five-point plan that I call H-E-A-R-T. As I've pointed out earlier in this chapter, each of the letters—H-E-A-R-T—represents a different step designed to help lower your risk of developing cardiovascular disease or lowering your risk of a cardiac event if you already have one of the five critical risk factors: high blood pressure, physical inactivity, overweight or obese with a surfeit of abdominal fat, pre-diabetes or diabetes, and elevated LDL cholesterol and trig-lycerides combined with low HDL (good) cholesterol. These all are "risk factors" for a reason—people with all, some or any one of these risk factors are far more likely to suffer a heart attack, stroke, and other manifestations of cardiovascular disease.

After learning how to achieve an optimal number, which you'll read about in the subsequent chapters, I encourage you to incorporate each of the steps into your daily routine. Achieve all five numbers and you'll optimally protect your heart. You need to know your numbers and what to do to achieve optimal numbers. Along with knowing your optimal number, you'll learn what you can do that will help you achieve an ideal number without medical intervention. One caveat: If your number(s) is up consistently, then it may be advisable to seek medical intervention.

H—HEAL YOUR BLOOD PRESSURE

What is high blood pressure and why is it important?
How many people have high blood pressure?
What is a normal blood pressure?
How can I achieve normal blood pressure without medication?
When should I seek medical advice?

E—ENERGIZE FOR A STRONG, HEALTHY HEART

Why is exercise good for my heart?
How many people exercise regularly?
What type and for how long should I exercise?
How much is too much?
How can I adopt and maintain a routine?

A—ACT AGAINST FAT

Is obesity predetermined or inherited?

How many people are overweight or obese?

What is a normal waist size?

Is body shape important?

What is visceral fat?

How can I achieve optimal waist size?

R—REDUCE BLOOD SUGAR

What is diabetes and why is it important?

How many are diagnosed with diabetes?

What is a normal blood sugar?

How can I achieve a normal blood sugar?

T—TACKLE TRIGLYCERIDES

What is high cholesterol and why is this important?

How many have high cholesterol?

What is normal cholesterol?

What can I do to lower my cholesterol without medication?

When should I seek medical advice?

These five numbers will never change. Following your H-E-A-R-T will always be needed, and achieving these five numbers will prevent heart disease. H-E-A-R-T is a reference and a guide to help you to achieve the five numbers. This is the "word." I didn't call this book *The Heart Health Bible* for nothing.

Often, I'm asked: "Why do I need to know these five numbers?" You need to know these numbers because millions of people are at risk of a cardiovascular event. Are you one of them? Wouldn't you like to know?

You may have risk factors such as family history, hypertension, high stress, obesity or a long history of smoking, but perhaps you're either too young or too symptom-free for your doctor to be concerned about your short-term heart attack risk.

Thanks to H-E-A-R-T, you're never too young or too healthy to find out if you're at risk for a cardiovascular event. Now you don't have to wait until there are any obvious signs of cardiovascular disease.

Along with MIRISK VP (for Myocardial Infarction Risk), and the Framingham Risk Score, long considered the gold standard of coronary risk assessment, H-E-A-R-T is not only great at identifying whether you're at immediate risk (in the next five years) and /or in jeopardy down the road, but it's the perfect tool to prevent a cardiovascular event from occurring in the first place.

WHY DO YOU NEED H-E-A-R-T?

Sometimes numbers don't tell the whole story. As an example, 50 percent of people who suffer a heart attack have "normal" cholesterol levels and many of those victims have no significant narrowing of their arteries. Using H-E-A-R-T, you can find in just a matter of minutes, where you stand today, and what you can to do to ensure a healthy future.

We'll never eliminate all heart disease. There are an entire category of inherited/genetic heart diseases that surface independent of our behaviors and lifestyle choices (though identifying these diseases can help slow their progression through preventative care). These include: hypertrophic, restrictive and dilated cardiomyopathies; inherited heart rhythm disorders such as LongQT and Brugada syndromes; familial cardiac amyloid; and inherited conditions that cause heart or heart-valve malformations. Following the pattern of a cardiac problem in your family can help your physicians predict the likelihood of you or other family members having the same condition. First, you need to figure out what your stress triggers are, learn to relax and reduce stress, then you need to exercise and eat right—an anti-inflammatory diet high in antioxidants.

Traditional risk assessment tools only consider short-term risk. H-E-A-R-T looks at long-term risk and prevention as well. Many people who are considered to be at low risk for cardiovascular disease in the short term are actually at high risk across their remaining lifespan. Children would fall into the category as an example.

Indeed, telling someone his/her short term is low is not ideal for a prevention model. Prevention doesn't have a beginning, middle, and end. There is no end to prevention. It's a lifestyle.

To eliminate the specter of cardiovascular disease from our lives we need to do everything in our power to prevent these risk factors from surfacing. I'd much rather get you to change your eating behavior than put in a stent or palliate your symptoms with medication. Always, it's preferable to engage in prevention than in the treating of existing risk factors. This is correct. Treating risk factors is thought of as secondary prevention. But for me, this doesn't go far enough. If I have to prescribe a statin or beta blocker, that means a horse or two is already out the barn door. If treating your existing hypertension means I can help lessen your risk and perhaps even avoid a coronary event, then I'm game, of course. No responsible physician would do otherwise. But why let it get to that point? Why not intervene early? Why spend hours chasing down a horse? Honestly, I don't want to treat obesity, diabetes, and hypertension—ever. That's a true prevention model. The focus of this book is primary prevention and that's not about fixing symptoms but preventing symptoms from ever appearing in the first place.

To avoid secondary prevention requires an entirely different level of commitment. It demands a change in the thinking and behaviors that led to hypertension, physical inactivity, overweight and obesity, insulin resistance and diabetes, and elevated cholesterol. Remember what the study concluded: Lifetime cardiovascular risks were "very low" with no risk factors but much higher with even one or two risk factors!

This is not to put down the Framingham Risk Score or MIRISK VP Assessment. These are wonderful tools that I use every day in my office. The Framingham Risk Score is a great way of looking ten years into the future to assess a person's cardiovascular disease risk. The MIRISK VP system, while not as widely used as the Framingham Risk Score, seems to be an even more accurate way to identifying folks at greatest risk for heart disease. The MIRISK VP test measures the blood levels of seven coronary artery disease-related proteins associated with plaque formation and inflammation, along with other clinical risk factors, such as family history, in an algorithm to determine an individual's personal risk of a cardiac event. The Framingham Risk Score doesn't pay attention to a person's family history—a significant drawback since family history plays a significant role in predicting heart disease.

But neither test takes other, less obvious variables into consideration. I know of no risk assessment tool that accounts for the stress brought on by family illness, the death of a loved one, job loss, or a failed marriage. To my knowledge, no test accounts for mood eating triggered by a depression, anxiety, a family argument or financial ruin. These tests are great at telling us our numbers, but as I'll repeat throughout this book, numbers only tell half the story. We all know that we should control our blood pressure, eat right, exercise more and manage stress. This is how we should behave. But how do we really behave? There's no assessment tool that accounts for that critical variable.

To make the real, lasting changes necessary to avoid a serious cardiac event we need to follow our H-E-A-R-T—an easy, accurate, and powerful method for accurately predicting your risk of a serious cardiac event and an important step on the road toward empowering you to take control of your cardiovascular health.

Although treating existing risk factors reduces a person's chances of heart disease, what's key is preventing them in adults for as long as possible through a heart-healthy lifestyle, which is more than eating healthy, exercising regularly, not smoking, and managing stress. Most important, it demands a change in thinking. Because it's only through a change in thinking, which changes the behavior that we will ever begin to gain ground and win the war against heart disease. It's time to follow your H-E-A-R-T!

Replacing maladaptive behaviors like overeating, physical inactivity, smoking, and drinking with the goal-oriented, action-focused techniques offered in this book are an effective way to achieve optimal heart health. Going forward, if you're feeling stressed, sitting down to eat, or while at work, remember to look at your hand and to recall how each of your fingers represents one of the 5 essential action steps discussed in this book. Hold up your hand and count: 1 is for heal your blood pressure, 2 is energize your heart, 3 is for act on fat, 4 is for reduce your blood sugar, and 5 is for tackle your triglycerides.

PART II

Understanding H-E-A-R-T... and Living It

CHAPTER 3

Heart of the Matter: Metabolic Syndrome

In this chapter I explain that cardiovascular disease rarely occurs as an isolated condition. Indeed, four major illnesses—hypertension, high triglycerides/high LDL cholesterol, abdominal obesity, and insulin resistance—appear together so frequently that they form a constellation of physical conditions and symptoms known as *Metabolic Syndrome* or *Syndrome X*. The tricky thing about *Metabolic Syndrome* is that it's not a disease—it's a syndrome. All syndromes are combinations of specific physical conditions and symptoms that occur together, and are related to each other. In this case, they're related to disorders in metabolism—how our body transforms food into energy. *Metabolic Syndrome* changes are profound—blood sugar shoots up, insulin levels rise, triglycerides and bad fats in the blood increase, good cholesterol drops, and blood thickens increasing the likelihood of blood clots, blood pressure spikes and blood vessels become inflamed. The bad news: Each of these symptoms independently is a risk factor for cardiovascular disease. Of course, the more risk factors you have, the greater the risk of a cardiovascular event. This chapter isn't meant to scare you. Rather, enlightenment is the emphasis. *Metabolic Syndrome* is treatable. In fact, it's often entirely reversible. But here's the catch: It's up to you. No one can do it for you. There is no drug that will do it. You have the power to reverse the course of *Metabolic Syndrome*.

THE MYSTERY AILMENT: PAUL'S STORY

"Practice medicine long enough and I guarantee that you'll come across some mysterious disease that defies treatment and will have you scratching your head," said one of my favorite professors in medical school. Wise words I've never forgotten. Think about it: Rheumatologists wrestle with fibromyalgia. Neurologists still don't have an effective treatment for chronic migraine headaches. Psychiatrists don't know all of the genes that play a role in the development of schizophrenia. Oncologists don't have an effective diagnostic tool for catching pancreatic cancer in its earliest stages, though I'm happy to report that as I wrote these words, an intrepid sixteen-year-old high school student may have solved that problem. For every step we take forward, we take two steps back.

It was maybe three years ago that I first encountered Paul, a rugged, handsome 45-year-old and former Australian Rules football player. Paul had moved to the U.S. a decade earlier for work. I got to know Paul after admitting him to the cardiac monitoring unit late one night when I was on call. Here was this big, burly guy lying in bed, clutching his chest, and looking very uncomfortable. He told me he had been experiencing intermittent chest pain that got worse when he exerted himself, which he did frequently as the CEO of a small but successful excavation company. Paul's EKG and blood tests came back normal, even his cholesterol seemed to be in check. But Paul's angina, and his description of its onset, put me on edge. It was something I couldn't summarily dismiss. I ordered a coronary angiogram.

That also came back negative. Paul's coronary arteries were as smooth as a baby's bottom. I couldn't find an obstruction with a fine, tooth comb. Angina and atherosclerotic plaque in the large coronary arteries that supply blood to the heart usually go hand in hand, like flipsides of the same coin. But there's another group of angina sufferers that have normal angiograms. Their chest pain mimics angina but they have healthy looking arteries, like Paul. I suspected that Paul had metabolic syndrome X, which we now know as metabolic syndrome. This would explain a lot since syndrome X was thought to be a "small coronary artery disease," meaning that it couldn't be detected using an angiography. That would explain the chest pain, which would stem from obstructed blood flow in small rather than large arteries.

The other strange thing about Paul's condition was his cholesterol numbers. His LDL (bad) cholesterol was 101, right around the ideal range. His total cholesterol was 192, which pleased me since anything below 200 is considered "desirable." But looking at Paul, who at 6'2" and 300 pounds was clearly obese, I thought we might be looking at these numbers through rose-colored glasses. In medicine, gross numbers seldom tell the whole story. Since Paul had other obvious risk factors for cardiovascular disease, I knew that I needed to dig a little further. What Paul's otherwise ideal numbers weren't telling me was the size of his LDL cholesterol particles. What do I mean by this? A person can have perfectly healthy cholesterol numbers but have hundreds, if not thousands of small LDL particles floating around his arteries, a very dangerous condition since small particles are easily oxidized and can penetrate the inner lining of the artery walls, leading to the development of atherosclerosis. LDL cholesterol does its damage by penetrating the endothelium, or inner lining of artery walls. Small LDL particles increase the risk of CAD even when overall LDL counts are at ideal levels. I ordered a nuclear magnetic resonance image test, which would give me a count of the number of LDL particles in Paul's blood. Higher counts indicate smaller particles. Paul came back with a thousand small particles. Insulin resistance causes these small particles.

The news just kept getting worse for Paul. His blood test also revealed high levels of Lp(a), or lipoprotein A, and a genetic cousin of LDL cholesterol. A high level of Lp(a) is a significant risk factor for the premature development of fatty deposits in arteries. Though Lp(a) isn't fully understood, it may interact with substances found in artery walls and contribute to the buildup of fatty deposits.

Things didn't stop there. Paul's weight and height left him with a BMI 38.5, meaning he was medically obese. His waist-to-hip ratio was 1.15—normal is less than 0.9 for men. His *fasting* plasma blood glucose level was a 106 mg/dl, indicating he had type 2 diabetes. This cluster of disorders led me to one conclusion: Paul had metabolic syndrome X.

Diagnosing Paul actually proved to be the easy part. What was far more challenging was explaining metabolic syndrome to him. If I diagnose a patient with unstable angina or atherosclerosis, they might be worried or alarmed but they at least understand what I'm talking about. Really, it's simple because angina and atherosclerosis are definable diseases. But when I told Paul he didn't have a single illness but rather a cluster of risk factors that were predisposing him to cardiovascular disease, not to mention a host of other conditions, he didn't seem to get it. "I'm not sure what you're telling me Dr. Kennedy. Do I have an illness, phobia, or disorder? And if I don't have an identifiable disease does that mean I'm a hypochondriac? Or, am I just plain nuts?"

After reassuring Paul that he wasn't "nuts," I gave him my standard spiel. After years of practicing medicine, I had my explanations down to a finely honed science. I told Paul that a syndrome is set of symptoms or conditions that consistently occur together and act both dependently and independently to suggest the presence of a certain disease or an increased chance of developing that disease. On the other hand, a disease or illness is a literal, diagnosed impairment of health or a condition of abnormal functioning such as atherosclerosis or diabetes.

Paul seemed to get it and assured me he'd take the steps necessary to reduce the cluster of risk factors that were predisposing him to a lifetime's worth of ill health.

A DISEASE WITH MANY FACES (DISEASE THAT WEARS MANY HATS)

Though Paul left the hospital the following day feeling better and fully committed to "turning things around" as he put it, I felt vaguely unsatisfied with our conversation. I understand that life is messy. Even things that appear quick and easy seldom are. But the great paradox of my life is that as a scientist, I crave a certain amount of order and certainty. My profession demands it. I need to provide patients with clear, cogent explanations.

Metabolic syndrome is one of those illnesses that screws up my predilection for explaining scientific concepts in clear, comprehensible language. Even Dr. Gerald Reaven, the esteemed Stanford University professor and researcher who coined the term "Metabolic Syndrome" in 1988 after he presented evidence showing the effect of an array of changes stemming from a then little known medical disorder called insulin resistance, fumbled a bit for clear, comprehensible explanation.

Dr. Reaven described metabolic syndrome as a "deadly heart ailment [that] begins in the blood stream shortly after we eat." Labeling carbohydrates as the primary culprit in the metabolic syndrome drama, Dr. Reaven went on to say that the glucose from these carbohydrates provides the energy our cells need to perform their many tasks. Whatever is left over is guided to storage cells by insulin, a protein secreted by the pancreas. "Insulin," said Dr. Reaven, "acts like a shepherd, herding its precious flock of sheep into the cellular 'corrals.'" Problems arise, he continued, when glucose behaves like "errant sheep, stubbornly refusing to go where the shepherd directs. When that happens, it's necessary for our bodies to send out more and more "shepherds" to get the "sheep" back into their homes." That many shepherds chasing thousands of sheep create a "prickly situation," say Dr. Reaven, "since they may tear up the field, ripping out or flattening down clumps of grass. Soon, the field that once looked so green and lush will be trampled and scarred, brown and dirty." A similar process happens in the human body in which glucose doesn't move into the storage cells at insulin's command, a phenomenon known as insulin resistance. When this happens, said Dr. Reaven, "the interior linings of our arteries, like the shepherd's grassy fields, get 'ripped' and 'trampled' while the body is trying to fix the problem. Eventually, the insulin "shepherds" corral the glucose, and order is restored in the body. But all is not well, for the playing field (the lining of your coronary arteries) has been compromised, and there's other damage, as well." This vastly damaged landscape sets the stage for heart disease, Dr. Reaven concluded.[1]

Still confused? You're not alone. Metabolic syndrome isn't a complicated illness.

In the intervening twenty-five years since Dr. Reaven's paradigmatic discovery, metabolic syndrome has become one of the most challenging conditions facing modern medical science. Depending on who's talking, it's been estimated that anywhere from 32–47 percent of American adults have metabolic syndrome. And because the prevalence of metabolic syndrome increases with age—roughly 40 percent of people over sixty are affected—this number will surely go up as life expectancy rises. Though metabolic syndrome is ubiquitous, it still flies under the radar. It's not an attention grabber like cancer, heart disease or obesity.

And this fact yields a fascinating question: How is it possible that a disease that affects tens of millions of people, and yields such deadly consequences, gets so little face time? Part of the fault lies with medical science, which still favors clearly identifiable problems that can be easily treated with medication. The other problem with metabolic syndrome is just what its name implies. It's not a disease; it's a syndrome. It's not one specific thing but a hodgepodge of cardiovascular risk factors, including high blood pressure, high fasting blood sugar, abdominal obesity, low LDL (good) cholesterol level, and high triglyceride level. Thus, metabolic syndrome doesn't fit neatly into a box and resists easy classification.

From a physician's perspective, treating metabolic syndrome can drive you a little haywire. You're dealing with multiple problems, all independent conditions, yet all interrelated. It's like trying to put out four to five small fires in separate parts of the Empire State building. The embers would never go out completely. Moreover, it wouldn't be just one doctor but multiple specialists that are called in to put out these fires. A nephrologist might intervene early with the hypertension and diabetes, the biggest causes of renal failure. An endocrinologist would look after the diabetes. A pulmonologist or even an otolaryngologist might treat obstructive sleep apnea; a bariatric surgeon might be the ticket for a case of morbid obesity. A cardiologist could potentially have his hand in every cookie jar. In the final analysis, you could wind up with five independent specialists looking after five separate problems. That's what it's like to treat metabolic syndrome.

And the problem is even worse for patients. Imagine living with as many as five adverse health conditions that put you at risk for type 2 diabetes and heart disease. But that's exactly the scenario that millions of people find themselves in as I write these words.

WHAT THE HECK IS METABOLIC SYNDROME?

Let's start with the basics. The word "metabolic" refers to all biochemical processes that take place within living cells that involve the body's normal functioning. There are two main types of metabolic processes: Catabolic processes involve the breakdown of complex molecules from food into smaller units that can be used as building blocks for new molecules or to provide energy. Anabolic processes, on the other hand, involve the use of energy to build new chemicals that become components of cells. Enzymes tie these reactions together. Digestion is the most obvious example of a catabolic process; new bone growth and increases in muscle mass are examples of anabolic processes (where do you think "anabolic" steroids come from?). Combined, the two types of metabolic processes allow the transformation of raw materials, or nutrients into existing tissue.

With metabolic syndrome a number of risk factors disrupt these processes. Risk factors are traits, conditions, or habits that increase your chance of developing a disease. Independently, the presence of some or all of these risk factors tell us that a person's metabolism is off. In most instances of metabolic syndrome, insulin—the great hormone that regulates blood sugars—is out of whack. High insulin levels play a big role in the occurrence of abdominal fat, one of the greatest predictors of cardiovascular disease.

DO YOU HAVE METABOLIC SYNDROME?

RISK FACTOR	DEFINING LEVEL
Abdominal obesity (waist measurement)	Men: 40 in. (102 cm) or more Women: 35 in. (88 cm) or more
Triglycerides	150 mg/dL or higher, or taking medicine for high triglycerides
High-density lipoprotein (HDL) cholesterol	Men: Less than 40 mg/dL Women: Less than 50 mg/dL Or taking medicine for low HDL cholesterol
Blood pressure	130/85 mm Hg or higher, or taking medicine for high blood pressure
Fasting blood sugar	100 mg/dL or higher, or taking medicine for high blood sugar

Typically, people with metabolic syndrome are prodigious producers of fat since they don't use insulin properly, a condition known as insulin resistance, which describes a diminished ability of some of the cells to respond properly to insulin. One of insulin's most important jobs is to coax cells to take in or, more precisely, store glucose as fat. Insulin resistance happens when they resist this call to store. Our bodies react by producing more insulin to reign in or stabilize our blood glucose, which spikes after such a scenario. If this situation persists for too long, a condition known as "hyperinsulinemia," or too much insulin in the blood, ensues. Hyperinsulinemia challenges the body to use stored fat for energy. Of course, that fat has to go somewhere. Either we burn it off through exercise or diet; or it gets stored, most often around our middle.

Metabolic syndrome is diagnosed via a lipid panel—basically blood work—except that it has no way of measuring for the primary risk factor, abdominal fat. Scales can be misleading, as we'll discuss in Chapter 7. Waist circumference is still the best gage to see if you're taking in too many calories. Excess calories affect not only the waist circumference part of metabolic syndrome, but the four other conditions as well. Special Alert: *Abdominal fat is the single greatest indicator of metabolic syndrome.* Excess calories are stored as fat, which affects your triglyceride number. Thus, controlling your food intake could be the best way of avoiding metabolic syndrome.

Exercise also is critical. It's a good balancer for insulin resistance. Overeating causes a spike in insulin—it's the body's way of eliminating excess blood sugar. Exercise helps lower blood sugar without using insulin, making the body more responsive to normal insulin.

Exercise assists the muscles with glucose (blood sugar) absorption without the need for insulin. Muscles use glucose as fuel, so in theory any type of activity can bring blood sugar levels down. Exercise also helps the body use insulin more efficiently, which in turn, helps the body use more glucose. And if you don't think you have time for exercise, think again. It's been suggested that several short intensive workouts a week may help lower blood sugar levels for twenty-four hours and even help prevent post-meal blood sugar spikes in people with type 2 diabetes.[2]

METABOLIC RISK FACTORS

The five conditions described below are metabolic risk factors. You can have any one of these risk factors, but they tend to cluster together. Three or more metabolic risk factors are an indication of metabolic syndrome.

Large Waistline

Also known as abdominal obesity or the dreaded "apple shape." Abdominal obesity puts you at greater risk for heart disease than excess fat in other parts of the body, such as on the hips or thighs. It's not too difficult to distinguish excess belly fat from other sorts of body fat. People with metabolic syndrome most often have apple-shaped bodies in which they carry a lot of weight around their stomachs. Paradoxically, a pear-shaped body is one where more weight is carried around the hips and buttocks with a narrower waist. Men, as a rule, tend to carry more weight around the middle; women carry their weight in the hips and buttocks. As unsightly as the pear-shaped body may be, especially for women, it's in the lower risk category for developing diabetes and heart disease.

It's my view that the waist circumference guidelines of 40 inches for men and 35 for women are too high. They're well above European guidelines of <94 cm for men and <80 cm for women recommended by the International Diabetes Foundation's Guidelines (part of its consensus worldwide definition for metabolic syndrome). As a nation, we're so used to being fat that we start our definition of a large waistline at three inches higher than other countries. It's no surprise that we have higher rates of overweight and obesity rate than other countries, though the guidelines are only part of the reason.

Organization	Measurement used	Definition of abdominal obesity
American Heart Association, National Heart, Lung and Blood Institute (10)	Waist circumference	Women: > 88 cm (35 inches) Men: > 102 cm (40 inches)
International Diabetes Federation (11)	Waist circumference	Women: > 80 cm (31.5 inches) Men: > 90 cm (35.5 inches) *Different cut-points for different ethnic groups*
World Health Organization (12)	Waist-to-hip ratio	Women: > 0.85 Men: > 0.9

METABOLIC SYNDROME: BELLY VS. BONES

Abdominal fat is known to be a leading cause of metabolic syndrome. However, a team of researchers at the Yale University School of Medicine claim that other factors may weigh just as heavily. Specifically, insulin resistance in skeletal muscle could lead to alterations in energy storage, setting the stage for metabolic syndrome.

The researchers found that insulin resistance in skeletal muscle—stemming from the decreased ability of muscle to make glycogen, the stored form of carbohydrate from food energy—promotes an elevated pattern of fat in the bloodstream that underpins metabolic syndrome.

Using a magnetic resonance spectroscopy to measure the production of liver and muscle triglyceride (the storage form of fat) and of glycogen (the storage form of carbohydrate), the researchers were able to observe how nutrients were channeled in the body in both insulin resistant and insulin sensitive human subjects. Interestingly, the study subjects were

(continues)

(continued)

all young, lean, non-smoking, healthy individuals who were sedentary and matched for physical activity. Aside from insulin resistance in one subject, none of the other participants had any of the risk factors associated with metabolic syndrome.

The study findings led the researchers to conclude that metabolic syndrome is really a problem with energy storage. Insulin resistance in muscle changes this storage pattern. What also was fascinating about the results is that insulin resistance in these young, lean, insulin resistant people, was independent of abdominal obesity, suggesting that this abnormality develops as metabolic syndrome progresses.

These are critical findings since having a better understanding of how insulin resistance alters energy storage before it leads to more serious problems can help prevent the onset of the metabolic syndrome, particularly in those most susceptible.

The best news the study found is that insulin resistance in skeletal muscle can be countered through a simple intervention: exercise.[3]

High Fasting Blood Sugar

Although it's a point of some contention, there is a general consensus that the two most important risk factors for cardiovascular disease associated with metabolic syndrome are abdominal or central obesity, and high blood sugar, which is the end product of insulin resistance. Both are the end game of eating too much, especially the sort of food found in the typical American diet. Our body compensates for excess blood sugar by overproducing insulin. It's a great quick fix, but continued overconsumption numbs the body to insulin's message, leading to the "resistance" part of insulin resistance. Avoiding insulin resistance is critical because it's the root cause of most cases of type 2 diabetes, a rapidly growing, yet almost entirely avoidable illness that stems from lifestyle-dependent risk factors, such as overweight/obesity, reduced physical activity, and an unhealthy diet. Even chronic, mildly high blood sugar is often an early sign of diabetes.

High Blood Pressure

In high school biology class, most of us learned that blood pressure is the force of blood pushing against the walls of our arteries as our hearts pumps blood. But if blood pressure stays high over time, it can damage the heart, leading to the build-up of artery clogging plaque. Blood pressure rises as our hearts labor to pump blood through increasingly narrow arteries. And hypertension is truly a silent killer, as few people show any outward signs or symptoms. In all likelihood this has much to do with its progression, as hypertension typically develops over many years. And hypertension is ubiquitous, affecting an alarming sixty-seven million American adults.[4] Like other metabolic risk factors, high blood pressure is frequently accompanied by abnormal cholesterol and blood sugar levels, which damage the arteries, kidneys, and heart. Fortunately, high blood pressure is easy to detect and treat, and as we'll see in Chapter 6, most people can keep their blood pressure in the normal, healthy range simply by adopting simple lifestyle changes.

Low HDL Cholesterol

HDL cholesterol is called "good" cholesterol for good reason—it's a biological scavenger, helping scrape away "bad" LDL cholesterol from your arteries. From there, HDL brings the excess cholesterol back to the liver, where it's broken down. Low HDL cholesterol accelerates the development of atherosclerosis because it impairs this cholesterol transport mechanism (low HDL may also lessen its protective effects, such as decreased oxidation of other lipoproteins). It's believed that low HDL cholesterol—known medically as hypoalphalipoproteinemia—is the most common metabolic syndrome risk factor in heart failure. Worst of all: Lowering LDL cholesterol might not be enough to avoid the risk of heart disease. HDL is considered low when its concentration in the blood is less than 40 mg/dL in men or less than 50 mg/dL in women.

High Triglyceride Level

Fat in our body is stored in the form of triglycerides, which is how we use them for energy—their primary function. But high triglyceride levels increase the risk for cardiovascular disease by making our blood thicker and stickier, meaning it's more likely to form clots. Elevated triglycerides alone can increase the risk of cardiovascular disease up to 14 percent in men, and 37 percent in women. *When combined with other risk factors, such as low HDL, high triglycerides increased the risk of heart disease by 32 percent in men and 76 percent in women!*[5] Obesity, poorly controlled diabetes, kidney disease, overeating coupled with physical inactivity, and excess alcohol consumption all lead to elevated triglycerides.

Age, hormone disorders such as polycystic ovary syndrome—an imbalance of sex hormones—family history of type 2 diabetes, history of gestational diabetes, and race and ethnicity all play a role and increase the risk for metabolic syndrome.

ETHNICITY AND METABOLIC SYNDROME

Ask anyone to describe my patient Flora and "hardworking" and "determined" always seemed to be the first two words that came to mind. Eighteen-hours days were not uncommon for this forty-four-year-old Latino woman. Most mornings, she was up before dawn, preparing lunches for her two children before taking them to school. For more than a week, Flora had been waking up with blurred vision, which she immediately attributed to her regular 5:30 AM wake up time and chronic lack of sleep.

When things didn't improve, Flora grew concerned. She'd suffered from type 2 diabetes, for which she was taking Metformin, an oral an-

(continues)

(continued)

tidiabetic drug. Flora also was overweight and had high blood pressure, neither of which she did anything about. Flora had a friend drive her to a local emergency room. Given Flora's recent medical history, the attending physician suspected her blurred vision might be the result of "diabetic retinopathy," a complication of diabetes that leads to blindness. The doctor performed a dilated eye exam, in which he placed drops in her eyes that opened her pupils to get a better view of her eyes. He noticed abnormal blood vessels, swelling and mild bleeding in the vitreous, the clear, jelly-like substance that fills the center of the eye. The doctor also performed a test known as a fluorescein angiography, which takes a detailed picture of the inside of the eye and allowed him to better pinpoint blood vessels that might be closed, broken down or leaking fluid.

Sitting in an exam room following her rests, the doctor started questioning Flora about her family medical history. She began to cry when she remembered her late mother, who died suddenly in her sleep late last year in her home country of Cuba. She recalled how she couldn't attend her mother's funeral because she could not afford to travel.

Flora's mentioned that her sisters attributed their mother's death to "old age," and never considered the true cause, which she later learned was coronary artery disease. The doctor suggested a battery of tests, particularly after learning of Flora's medical history and her recent medical problems. When the results came back a few days later, Flora learned that not only did she have diabetes and hypertension, but also her LDL cholesterol was 195 md/dL, putting her in the "very high" risk category. When Flora visited the doctor a few days later he was blunt. "Flora, you have metabolic syndrome. As of now, you're at great risk of a stroke or heart attack."

Flora knew that she had health problems but didn't realize that things were so bad. Of course, Flora was not alone. Across the board, minority women in particular are less likely than white women to be aware of the risks and symptoms of heart disease. And even when they are aware, they are less likely to try to reduce their risks or seek treatment.[6] The great irony of these findings is that minority women generally have a greater

(continues)

(continued)

number of cardiovascular health risks than any other demographic group. More than 80 percent of African-American and 70 percent of Hispanic women are overweight or obese, compared to just 50 percent of white women. They also show that a mere 10 percent of minority women have physically active lifestyles and tend to suffer from high blood pressure and diabetes in record numbers.[7,8] Although a comparatively small percentage of Hispanic women like Flora suffer from heart disease, they tend to develop symptoms a full decade earlier than white women.

Part of the problem is that there are not enough studies focusing on minority women. Moreover, there aren't enough programs that deliver heart-healthy information to minority and lower income women. Thus, there's something of a knowledge gap of their underlying risks and how we can decrease those risks.

Through a combination of medication, and a heart-healthy lifestyle that included better food choices, and cutting back on her hours at work, Flora was able to avert disaster.

Six months later I saw Flora in my office. She looked amazing. Her smile beaming and she had noticeably lost weight. I remember her first words to me were, "Thank you for the life preserver. Look, doc, it fits!" She took a red and white life preserver from behind the examining room table, slipped it over her head and let it rest on her hips, proving her waist size had significantly shrunken. Flora had traded her spare tire for a life preserver.

One year prior to this meeting I told Flora that when she committed to the lifestyle and followed her H-E-A-R-T that she would begin to lose weight in her mid-section. I explained how this visible external change correlated with positive internal changes with her blood pressure, cholesterol, and blood sugar. She said to me, "So I have to lose my spare tire?" And I responded, "Yes Flora, when you can fit through a doughnut like life preserver, you'll know you are there."

I left the room thinking what a powerful metaphor this was and how Flora's life preserver was her commitment to following her H-E-A-R-T.

TAKING A BITE OUT OF METABOLIC SYNDROME

Cleary, the treatment and ultimately the prevention of metabolic syndrome focuses on smart lifestyle choices. But that's sometimes easier said than done. As doctors, I don't think we do a good enough job communicating about the risks associated with having metabolic syndrome. It's incumbent upon us better explain to patients exactly what having metabolic syndrome means in terms of developing diabetes and heart disease.

Patients also need to get on board. Not simply by knowing their risk factors, but in focusing on the behaviors that led them to develop these risk factors in the first place. It's one thing to know that metabolic syndrome can be averted or even prevented with better lifestyle choices. It's another matter to create the conditions that allow those changes to be put into place. That requires a whole new level of commitment that goes beyond superficial lifestyle changes.

HOW H-E-A-R-T CAN HELP

Patients also need to get on board. Not simply in knowing their risk factors, but also on targeting the behaviors that led them to develop these risk factors in the first place. It's one thing to understand that metabolic syndrome can be averted or even prevented with better lifestyle choices. It's another matter to create the conditions that allow those changes to be put into place. That requires a whole new level of commitment that goes beyond changing your waistline or exercising more.

I think that our understanding and discovery of the metabolic syndrome may be the most important research in the last fifty years in cardiology because being overweight and obese is visible and tangible. On the other hand, you can't always see or feel your blood pressure, blood sugar, or cholesterol level, though I've found that

MEASURING YOUR WAIST SIZE

How to measure your waist circumference: Places a tape measure snugly around your bare abdomen just above your hip bones. Exhale. Then take the measurement.

Source: National Institutes of Health, *The Practical Guide: Identification, Evaluation, and Treatment of Overweight and Obesity in Adults.*

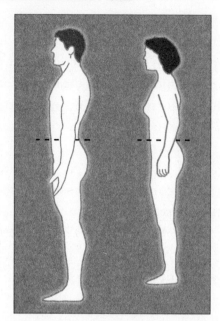

once patients understand the correlation between their body size and the internal storm it creates, they are more apt to change and maintain their H-E-A-R-T.

CHAPTER 4

Blood Pressure:
Your Heart Under Pressure

In this chapter you'll learn the first step to follow your heart by "H—healing your blood pressure."

Imagine falling asleep one night thinking you were in perfectly good health, only to wake up the next morning to find the opposite was true. That sort of frightening revelation happened for roughly forty-five million Americans less than a decade ago after the National Heart, Lung, and Blood Institute (NHLBI) released new guidelines for the prevention, detection, and treatment of high blood pressure. Today, an estimated fifty million Americans live with high blood pressure.[1] While we spend billions annually on medication, the death rate from hypertension keeps rising, thirty-six percent in the past decade alone. When hypertension touches lives, as it has for nearly every adult American in some fashion, it can be frightening and confusing. Because high blood pressure shows few outside symptoms, it often flies under the radar, even when readings reach dangerously high levels. It's estimated that 28 percent of Americans have high blood pressure and don't know it! But make no mistake: It's killing us. Though high blood pressure is an independent risk factor for cardiovascular disease and stroke, it's one of the easiest to prevent and can almost always be controlled without medication. This chapter gives you a firm grip on the tools needed control their blood pressure, including an inside look at my BREATHE™ Technique, the surest and quickest way to reign in blood pressure naturally.

CHRIS'S STORY

Young, healthy, and a successful attorney and accomplished amateur triathlete, Chris, was literally racing through life. One day, at the age of forty-five, Chris was doing what a lot of lawyers do every day. He was sitting in court with a client who was in the midst of a messy and costly divorce. The client, a successful software developer and angel investor, had built up a small empire but now was in danger of losing it all, including custody of his children, to a vengeful ex-wife, whose only goal seemed to be extracting as much flesh as possible from her estranged husband. Predictably, Chris soon found himself caught in a vicious cycle of internalizing and absorbing his client's drama and emotional distress. Chris had spent hours on this case, often working late into the night, missing his son's baseball games, his daughter's dance recitals, and date nights with his wife, which contributed to his own bit of marital discord.

As the case wore on, with no settlement in sight, Chris noticed his meetings with his client were becoming more and more stressful, but he attributed this to "normal pressure." One day while he walking up the courthouse stairs to file a motion for his client, he felt something in his chest. Then, without warning, he lost complete control of his right hand. Chris had never experienced anything like this before. Chris rarely thought about his health, save for an annual checkup. After all, he was never sick and had recently completed his third half marathon. He quickly brushed off this "incident," frantically gathered his documents, grabbed his briefcase, and dashed off to the courtroom.

Just as he approached the stand to confer with the judge, things took a sudden and frightening turn for the worse. He couldn't speak. His mouth was moving but no words were coming out. He tried motioning for help but could barely raise his arms. A clerk, who'd lost his mother years earlier to a stroke, recognized what was happening, rushed over and immediately dialed 911. He helped Chris, who was now having trouble standing, out of the courtroom. Paramedics arrived quickly and within minutes Chris was lying on a stretcher. They informed Chris that he had accelerated hypertension, meaning his blood pressure was through the roof and measured a whopping 240/140 mm Hg (120/80 is considered optimal). At the hospital, doctors ordered a CT and MRI, which revealed a hemorrhagic stroke, which occurs when a blood vessel in the brain breaks or ruptures. High blood pressure and brain aneurysms are the two leading causes of hemorrhagic stroke, the number three cause of death in the U.S. and a leading cause of disability. Bleeding had flooded the parts of Chris's brain involved with movement and speech, which explained his difficulties in court.

Chris was transferred to the intensive care unit, where doctors inserted a breathing tube since bleeding in the brain can cause breathing to stop or become irregular. For five days, doctors monitored Chris's blood pressure, and he was given drugs to control swelling and an anti-seizure medication. A second CT scan revealed hydrocephalus, which is the buildup of fluid within the brain. To correct this condition, Chris's doctors performed an endoscopic ventriculostomy, a procedure to drain the fluid and reduce the risk of a second stroke. Two days after the procedure, Chris spoke with his doctors. "You're lucky we caught this before there was too much damage. The risk of stroke is directly related to how high the blood pressure is," they told him.

How could something like a stroke strike an otherwise healthy young man? How does high blood pressure cause a stroke? High blood pressure can weaken the walls of the tube like structures that carry oxygen to the brain. The pressure inside these delicate tubes can lead to stretching, dilating and in some cases, as that of Chris, even bursting like a balloon over-filled with air. The extra blood from the bursting blood vessel then begins to accumulate and presses on brain structures, which compromises function. This type of stroke happens suddenly, within minutes, and is known as a "hemmorhagic" stroke.

Over time high blood pressure can damage the inner lining of the arteries, which can increase the risk of "atherosclerosis" a process that leads to a buildup of plaque on the vessel walls much like a coral reef. Eventually the plaque can obstruct blood flow and impair brain function and is known as an "ischemic" stroke. In the intervening six years since his stroke, Chris has fully recovered his abilities and still occasionally competes in races. Even more fortunately, this experience has changed Chris. As he told me recently, "I'm completely back to normal and feel fully recovered. But I don't feel like the same person I was before."

"What's different," I asked?

"My priorities have shifted. Before the stroke I was too career and 'me' oriented. I try to leave the office by 6 and I no longer work on weekends, even though that decision has cut into my bottom line. But now I have time for my family, which has been far more fulfilling than a few extra dollars or finishing in first place in a triathlon. It sounds weird but this experience has given me my life back."

WHAT IS HIGH BLOOD PRESSURE?

Blood pressure is like cholesterol—essential for life. And it's the one thing most of us know something about. If you've had a physical exam then you've had your blood pressure taken. Normal blood pressure is 120/80mmHg (see chart next page). When blood pressure exceeds these values we call it high blood pressure, or hypertension. Basically, high blood pressure creates resistance to the heart's ability to pump blood. Thus, the heart must work harder than normal to circulate blood through the blood vessels and to maintain that elevated blood pressure.

Clinically speaking, hypertension is defined as an elevated Systolic Blood Pressure, Diastolic Blood Pressure, or both. A clinical definition of hypertension is "The mean of two or more properly measured seated BP measurements taken on two or more occasions and are found to be above the normal value of 120/80 mmHg" according to guidelines from the American Heart Association. I know that sounds complicated but it's not that bad. Blood pressure is always is measured in two values, hence a reading of 120/80 mmHg. These two values equate to two types of blood pressure: systolic and diastolic. Using the example above, 120 is systolic blood pressure, and 80 is diastolic blood pressure. Systolic always comes before diastolic.

SYSTOLIC AND DIASTOLIC BLOOD PRESSURE

So what are these systolic and diastolic blood pressures? As long as we're alive, our heart never stops beating. Every time the heart beats, the pressure generated by the force of the heart when it pumps blood through the arteries is called the systolic blood pressure. Systolic blood pressure always is higher than diastolic blood pressure because the pressure of the contracting heart means that blood is being forced into the arteries, which are at a low pressure. If the pressure wasn't high, blood wouldn't be able to travel away from your heart against gravity and pressure. Of course, our arteries also are elastic, much like a long rubber tube. These rubber tubes stretch when the heart pumps blood into them. When the heart relaxes, the stretched

	Diastolic	Systolic
Definition:	It is the pressure that is exerted on the walls of the various arteries around the body in between heart beats when the heart is relaxed.	It measures the amount of pressure that blood exerts on arteries and vessels while the heart is beating.
Normal range:	60 – 80 mmHg (adults); 65 mmHg (infants); 65 mmHg (6 to 9 years)	90 – 120 mmHg (adults); 95 mmHg (infants); 100 mmHg (6 to 9 years)
Importance with age:	Diastolic readings are particularly important in monitoring blood pressure in younger individuals.	As a person's age increases, so too the importance of their systolic blood blood pressure measurement.
Blood Pressure:	Diastolic represents the minimum pressure in the arteries.	Systolic represents the maximum pressure exerted on the arteries.
Blood Pressure reading:	The lower number is diastolic pressure.	The higher number is the systolic. pressure.
Ventricles of the heart:	Fill with blood	Left ventricles contract
Etymology:	"Diastolic" comes from the Greek diastole meaning "a drawing apart."	"Systolic" comes from the Greek systole meaning "a drawing together or a contraction."
Blood Vessels:	Relaxed	Contracted

arteries contract back and then the arteries exert pressure on the blood. This pressure is called <u>diastolic blood pressure</u>—its value is always less than the systolic blood pressure (see chart).

HIGH BLOOD PRESSURE AND HYPERTENSION: ARE THEY ONE IN THE SAME?

It's a question I'm often asked since the two terms are used interchangeably. They are in fact different. High blood pressure is an increase in blood pressure; hypertension is a disease. Slight increase(s) in blood pressure is a normal part of daily life. We call this labile hypertension and it's best described as an episodic rise in blood pressure. When you exercise, raise your voice, or get excited before a big event such as a wedding, your heart beats faster, your pulse quickens, both of which combine to raise your blood pressure. This is a normal part of healthy living. It's how your body copes with everyday life events.

If your blood pressure remains continuously elevated, however, even while you're at rest, that's an indication that something is amiss. We define hypertension as three separate blood pressure recordings on three different days >140 systolic and >85 diastolic. This implies that blood pressure is persistently elevated and you've crossed the hypertension threshold.

WHY HYPERTENSION MATTERS

High Blood Pressure is known as the "silent killer" for good reason—it's a major risk factor for many dreaded medical conditions. Even a moderate raise in arterial blood pressure can shorten life expectancy. Hypertension, as mentioned above, puts your heart under continuous stress. This weakens your heart and in the long run can lead to various heart diseases. You should never forget this because death from heart attacks is the leading cause of death today.

Unfortunately, this silent killer strikes at more than one point. Hypertension not only negatively affects your heart but also damages your kidneys, eyes, blood vessels, and brain. These are the major organs of your body, and having hypertension puts your life at risk from damage to these organs. There are other minor adverse effects as well. These give us reason enough to be highly concerned about maintaining our blood pressure in the normal range—which would remove all the stress on these organs. Fortunately, this silent killer can be tamed. Hypertension can be easily managed with proper guidance and the techniques I offer at the end of this chapter.

SIGNS AND SYMPTOMS

The irony of hypertension is that while it's a potentially life-threatening situation it's usually not accompanied by any overt signs or symptoms (hence, the "silent killer" moniker). But symptoms develop when your blood pressure escalates beyond the point where your body can tolerate it. When this happens, most people with high blood pressure report some or even all of these symptoms:

1. Headaches (particularly at the back of the head and in the morning)
2. Lightheadedness
3. Dizziness
4. Tinnitus (buzzing or ringing in the ears)
5. Altered vision
6. Fainting episodes

ALL HYPERTENSIONS ARE NOT CREATED EQUAL

If you're diagnosed with hypertension, that doesn't mean you're destined for a lifetime of daily medication. Like many illnesses, doctors divide hypertension into stages. The Joint National Commission for hypertension, or JNC-7, classify hypertension into the following five stages:

1. **Normal BP**: Up to but not exceeding 120/80 mmHg
2. **Pre-Hypertension Stage 1**: 120–140/80–90 mmHg
3. **Pre-Hypertension Stage 2**: 140–160/90–100 mmHg
4. **Hypertension**: Above 160/100 mmHg

This is the stage when you need to take action and may need to aggressively combat hypertension with prescription medicines due to a high risk of organ damage.

5. Hypertensive Crisis: Above 200/110 mmHg

This is an emergency situation and can lead to potentially life threatening situations including a heart attack and stroke. The patient should been seen immediately by a doctor.[2]

The main reason behind this classification is that you do not need to start taking prescription medicines immediately. The JNC-7 suggests that people with pre-hypertension do not need heavy medication. They can bring their BP back to normal through lifestyle modifications, which I list in this chapter.[3]

This suggestion is for people who are healthy otherwise. Elderly people or people who have other major diseases like diabetes or heart diseases should always take medication no matter what stage of hypertension they have. This is a critical health and safety consideration.

THE MANY FACES OF HYPERTENSION

1. Primary Hypertension or Essential Hypertension is the most common type of hypertension. This is form of the hypertension that does not have any identifiable cause.

2. Secondary hypertension is hypertension, which has a definite cause such as kidney disease or obesity.

3. Malignant hypertension often stems from *hypertensive crisis.* It is diagnosed when there is evidence of direct damage to one or more organs as a result of severely elevated blood pressure.

4. White Coat Hypertension. Some people experience high blood pressure when they see a doctor who is about to examine them. This is due to apprehension or the fear of the unknown. The patient is afraid what the doctor might say—whether or not they have some dreaded disease. This is known as *white coat hypertension* This situation usually resolves when the patient sits and relaxes for about 10 minutes.

5. Borderline Hypertension is the former word for what is now known as **Pre-Hypertension.** This stage reflects that you have hypertension developing in your system and you need to take measures now before you become Hypertensive and risk organ damage.

WHAT CAUSES HYPERTENSION?

The exact cause of high blood pressure varies from person to person. Factors and conditions contributing to the development of hypertension are:

1. Smoking
2. Excess Weight or Obesity
3. Lack of physical activity
4. Sedentary lifestyle
5. High Salt Intake
6. High Alcohol Consumption (more than 1 to 2 drinks per day)
7. 65 or older
8. Genetics
9. Family history of high blood pressure
10. Chronic kidney disease
11. Adrenal and thyroid disorders
12. Medications that constrict blood vessels
13. High Cholesterol
14. Artherosclerosis—Narrowing of arteries due to high lipid content in the body
15. Stress
16. Thyroid problem
17. Genetics—Family history of high blood pressure
18. Race—African-Americans are at higher risk of developing hypertension
19. Pregnancy
20. Birth control pills—specifically those containing estrogen
21. Age—above thirty-five years

Kidney disease ranks highest as the cause of secondary hypertension because our kidneys need pressure to filter the blood. So they have the ability to increase blood pressure when they are not functioning properly due to tumors or other abnormalities that cause the adrenal glands (small glands present on top of the kidneys) to secrete excess amounts of the hormones that elevate blood pressure.

Essential hypertension is greatly influenced by diet and lifestyle. The link between salt and high blood pressure is especially compelling. People living on the northern islands of Japan eat more salt per capita than anyone else in the world and have the highest incidence of essential hypertension. By contrast, people who add no salt to their food show virtually no traces of essential hypertension.

THINGS TO BE WORRIED ABOUT—TAKE IMMEDIATE ACTION TO BE SAFE FROM THESE DANGERS!

Hypertension can really damage your body in the long run—if worrying makes you take action then you should definitely worry because hypertension, if untreated, can result in following:

Damage to arteries—Continuously raised high blood pressure can damage the cells of your arteries' inner lining. This causes arteriosclerosis—or hardening of the arteries—which can lead to serious cardiovascular complications.

Damage to the heart—Uncontrolled high blood pressure can damage your heart in a number of ways, such as:

1. Coronary artery disease. Coronary artery disease affects the arteries that supply blood to your heart muscle. Arteries narrowed by coronary artery disease don't allow blood to flow freely through your arteries. When blood can't flow freely to your heart, it can cause chest pain, irregular heart rhythms (arrhythmias), and heart attack.

2. Enlarged left heart. High blood pressure forces your heart to work harder than necessary in order to pump blood to the rest of your body. This causes the left ventricle (the part of the heart which pumps blood to your body) to thicken and grow abnormally. Medically this is known as Left Ventricular Hypertrophy. This condition increases the risk of heart failure and can cause continuous cough because the enlarged heart now presses against the lung.

3. Heart failure. Over time, the stress on your heart caused by high blood pressure weakens the heart muscle and it works less efficiently. This eventually leads to heart failure—which is simply when the heart cannot maintain balance between the demand and supply of blood.

Brain Damage can result from Hypertension.

1. Transient ischemic attack or **TIA** results when the brain's blood supply is restricted due to narrowing of the arteries by atherosclerosis or blood clot (both of which can arise from high blood pressure). If not resolved, this can lead to brain damage.

2. Stroke—High blood pressure damages and weakens the brain's blood vessels, causing them to rupture or leak. People with high blood pressure sometimes get headaches because the delicate vessels in the brain cannot handle such high pressure of blood. When this pressure becomes too much, they get ruptured and leak blood, which can clog up to form clots and block other blood vessels. This results in brain hemorrhage and stroke, which can be fatal.

3. Dementia or loss of memory can result from interruption of blood flow to the brain due to stroke or TIA, both of which may be caused by high blood pressure.

4. Damage to Kidneys or Kidney failure. High blood pressure can damage both the large arteries leading to your kidneys and the tiny blood vessels (glomeruli) within the kidneys. As a result your kidneys cannot effectively filter waste from your blood. This leads to accumulation of dangerous levels of fluid and poisonous waste in your blood, which may require dialysis or kidney transplantation.

HEALING HYPERTENSION: HOW H-E-A-R-T CAN HELP

A diagnosis of hypertension is indeed a major concern. But I would also caution you not to over worry because here we will educate you about hypertension and tell you how to live a healthy and hypertension-free life. With strong will and proper guidance you don't have to worry about high blood pressure ever again (unless you get stuck visiting your in-laws). Dietary and lifestyle changes can improve blood pressure control and decrease the risk of associated health complications. Although drug treatment is recommended for people for whom lifestyle changes prove ineffective or insufficient. I recommend the following lifestyle modifications for people with pre-hypertension as well as hypertension:

1. Weight reduction. Maintain a normal weight with a target body mass index (BMI) of 18.5 to 24.9. This can result in an approximate reduction in systolic blood pressure of 5–20 points per 10 kilograms of weight loss, according to the JNC-7.

2. 5 for 1 Diet. If you're looking for a dietary approach to heal hypertension, consider an eating plan rich in fruits, vegetables, and low-fat dairy products. Reduce saturated and total fat. This can be expected to drop systolic blood pressure by 8–14 points.

3. Lower Salt Intake. Reduce dietary sodium to less than 2,400 milligrams or about 1 teaspoon a day. According to the JNC-7, a DASH eating plan limiting salt intake to 1,600-milligram has effects similar to a single drug therapy. The approximate reduction in blood pressure would be 2–8 points.

4. Aerobic Physical Activity. Engage in regular physical activity, such as brisk walking for at least 30 minutes per day. This can decrease systolic blood pressure by 4–9 points.

5. Moderation of Alcohol Consumption. Men should limit alcohol intake to no more than two drinks per day. The type of alcohol defines a standard drink. A standard drink, such as a 12-ounce bottle of beer, a 5-ounce glass of wine, or 1.5-ounce shot of 80-proof distilled spirits, has between 11 and 14 grams of alcohol. Limiting the amount of alcohol to this quantity is expected to result in a reduction in systolic blood pressure by 2–4 points. This also protects your liver and kidneys from damage.

6. Hypertension Medications should be taken in conjunction along with an attempt to reduce the causes of high blood pressure.

CAN YOU BREATHE AWAY HYPERTENSION?

BREATHE™ is an acronym for a relaxation technique I created to help heal hypertension. For best results, I suggest you follow the simple step-wise template below. Remember that conscious breathing connects the heart and brain, creating dialogue between these two organs. Each of the letters in the word BREATHE™ has special significance and represents one of the seven steps that comprise the technique. Follow each step closely and apply them to the exercises that follow.

B in B-R-E-A-T-H-E is for the beginning.
Begin your exercise each day at a time and place that fits best with your lifestyle. Whatever time or place you choose, don't force the issue. This technique should help. Thus, it shouldn't feel forced or seem like a chore. I have a patient, a truck driver in fact, who practices early morning on a loading dock just before checking his inventory and planning his daily delivery route. A surgeon colleague I know practices at a scrub

(continues)

(continued)

sink just prior to operating, a practice made famous by Mehmet Oz. If you work in a busy office, consider a short walk to a quiet place such as a park during your lunch hour. If that's not possible, close your office door and shut off the phone. Most of my patients who practice BREATHE™ do so right after they wake up, which they say gives them focus and helps them achieve their daily goals. Others use BREATHE™ right before bedtime, which I've noticed helps calm the mind, leading to better quality sleep. Wherever or whenever you decide to use BREATHE™, pick a location where you won't be interrupted for fifteen minutes, which is the amount of time needed to develope a rhythm, routine, gain mastery and optimize results. Finally, remember to start the BREATHE™ journey with a positive attitude. Turn the next fifteen minutes is a well-deserved gift to yourself.

R in B-R-E-A-T-H-E is for relaxation.

It may seem counterintuitive but it takes work to relax! I'm not talking about diving into a beanbag chair, flipping on the TV, and ripping open a bag of chips. The type of relaxation needed for BREATHE™ requires concentration, focus and conscious breathing. To start, clear your mind of all thoughts. Concentrate only on your breath. Recall what I said earlier: focused, controlled and conscious breathing establishes a dialogue between the heart and brain. A helpful imagery tool is something I call the *Path to Relaxation and Flow*. Imagine a beautiful hiking path. Each step you take along the path allows you to become more relaxed. The reward for completing each step along the path always is the same—a peaceful and serene oasis at the foot of the majestic flowing river.

Conscious Breathing

First, sit in a comfortable chair with armrests. Your body should be as relaxed as possible, so allow the weight of your arms and legs to feel

(continues)

(continued)

supported by the chair. Your feet should rest comfortably on the ground. Now focus on your breathing. To begin, place one hand on a part of your chest or preferably your abdomen. Watch your hand rise and fall with each breath. Inhale and exhale through your nose if possible, a technique known in yogic circles as *ujjayi breath*. If you're congested or are just unable to breathe through your nose, your mouth will suffice.

Inhale deeply and slowly through your nose and "feel" the breath as it moves into your abdomen. You'll see and sense your abdomen rising with each inhalation. Your chest, on the other hand, should move only slightly. Exhale through your mouth, keeping your mouth, tongue, and jaw relaxed. If possible, extend your exhalation for a count of seven, like the number of letters in the word BREATHE™.

Relax, focusing only on the sound and feeling of those slow deep breaths.

You might detect the subtle conversation between your heart and brain. As you take in a breath, you may notice your pulse increases slightly as you exhale, while your heart rate simultaneously decreases.

Repeat this breathing series seven times. Done properly, it's my belief that you'll feel more relaxed. Once you feel all your muscles relax and your entire weight supported by your chair, then you know it's time to move on to the next step in BREATHE™. Like any skill, conscious breathing gets easier with practice. In time, conscious breathing will become rote, allowing you to devote greater focus to the heart-healing guided imagery that comprises the second component of the BREATHE™ technique.

E in B-R-E-A-T-H-E is for envision.

Picturing the finish line or desired goal is a common practice in sports, business, and academics. Indeed, thought leaders at the world's most innovative and successful companies rely heavily on dreaming, imagining, and thinking outside the box. Without imagination we'd still be stuck on square 1. From medical science to wireless technology, all

(continues)

(continued)

significant breakthroughs are born out of an active imagination. Imagination has important applications for maintaining good health. When you practice BREATHE™, imagine each part of your heart healthy and strong. Patients with a thorough understanding of their medical condition and who use visualization have better overall health. Use the healing metaphors in exercises to soothe and calm your body and allow your heart to rest and idle. Visualize your heart as strong and powerful with all the parts working synergistically and efficiently. Remember that the special imagery exercises lower your heart rate, lower your blood pressure, and strengthen your immune system. Each time you perform these exercises visualize your heart and imagine all four parts—the arteries, muscle, valves, and electrical system. Analyze what they look like and how they work synergistically, nourishing every part of your body with a constant, unimpeded flow of blood.

Relaxation training using guided imagery has been shown to reduce cortisol output.

Research has shown that guided imagery may:
Reduce stress and anxiety
Decrease pain
Decrease side effects
Decrease blood pressure
Decrease blood glucose levels (Diabetes)
Decrease allergy and respiratory symptoms
Decrease the severity of headaches
Decrease hospital costs
Enhance bone and wound healing
Enhance sleep
Enhance self-confidence
Assist in losses (job, divorces, death)
Enhance quality of life

(continues)

(continued)

A in B-R-E-A-T-H-E is for apply.

When reading through the guided imagery exercises and observing the accompanying art, imagine how the heart-healing images and metaphors can be applied and relate to your healthy heart. Stay focused concentrating on the significance of the images because it is easy to get distracted.

Along the way, you may lose focus or feel a little anxious or frustrated. This is normal. Do not worry because getting back on track is easy. Use this as a reminder of the conversation. Apply the principles of this technique and recall that conscious breathing is the way back into the conversation and helps you refocus. The sensations and real physiological changes stress creates are reminders of the conversation and an invitation to stop stress in its tracks.

The *apply* step in BREATHE™ is a two-fold process. The first involves applying the meaning of the metaphors to an efficiently working heart. The second involves using the technique to help cope during stressful situations or feeling anxious or upset. With regular practice, you'll start to file away each heart-healing metaphor in your memory bank. In this way, they can be called upon whenever needed.

T in B-R-E-A-T-H-E is for treatment.

BREATHE™ is both a pleasurable and therapeutic exercise. The fifteen minutes you spend a day on BREATHE™ is a gift you give to yourself. It's the ultimate form of self-care. Remember as well that BREATHE™ isn't a chore, duty or errand to check off on your "to-do" list. Rather, it's an extremely pleasant and pleasurable endeavor that you will begin to look forward to. BREATHE™ is a treatment—like rewarding yourself with a massage or facial at a leading spa. The goal is an invigorated and relaxed body and mind.

H in B-R-E-A-T-H-E is for Heal.

BREATHE™ is healing. Why else would I suggest you do it? In as little as fifteen minutes a day, BREATHE™ can strengthen the neural net-

(continues)

(continued)

works that connect your heart and brain. You will consistently elicit the relaxation response, which has a number of healing physiological benefits including increased heart rate variability, decreased blood pressure, enhanced immune response, improved focus and lower pulse rate. BREATHE™ combines two proven relaxation techniques and can be used anytime and virtually anywhere. It is accessible to anyone and simple to learn. I'm convinced that the transformative healing properties of BREATHE™ will help you remain positive and focused.

E in B-R-E-A-T-H-E is for End.

Every effective exercise has a beginning, middle and end. Having successfully completed your exercises and carefully and mindfully embodied the heart-healing metaphors, you will hopefully feel more relaxed. However, you should also feel energized and revitalized—ready to take on any challenge. Actively concentrating on the rhythm and rate of your breathing increases the oxygen your blood carries to your tissues and internal organs, especially your heart.

Before finishing, make a checklist of the healing metaphors. Imagine how you use of these metaphors to help defuse a difficult situation.

Remember that the combined guided imagery and breath work exercises in each chapter were carefully crafted and are filled with heart-healing metaphors that relate to the properly functioning heart parts. Similar to the concept of Qi in Chinese medicine, the BREATHE™ exercises emphasize how flow relates to an efficient, healthy, and smoothly running cardiovascular system. BREATHE™ helps "unblock" heart parts and promotes flow in the electrical, valvular, muscular and arterial systems.

This simple, cost-effective technique has withstood the test of time and modern research shows many positive health benefits of its use. Guided imagery and breath work have been used successfully for reducing anxiety, improving coping skills, lowering blood pressure, and for de-

(continues)

(continued)

creasing post-operative pain. They have also been shown to have potent immune bolstering effects such as an increase in the number of natural killer cells, which are potent immune cells that help ward off infection. Relaxation therapies such as BREATHE™ have also been shown to lower levels of the stress hormone cortisol which in large amounts (like those seen with chronic stress) can weaken our body's ability to fight infection and slow tissue repair.

TAKE H-E-A-R-T

Hypertension is a medical disorder. Yet, as a chronic disease, it's also clearly a lifestyle disorder, aggravated in 90 percent of cases by unhealthy behaviors. As we've seen throughout this book, all behaviorally based illnesses start with our thinking. While we're able to control most cases of hypertension with medication, fixing the underlying behaviors that contribute to the majority of hypertension cases remains one of medicine's greatest challenges. As an editorial in the highly regarded *International Journal of Hypertension* points out, "Although there is clear consensus on the impact of behaviors such as exercise and nutrition on blood pressure, relatively little is known about how to motivate people to take up and consistently engage in these health behaviors." It's one thing to encourage people to change their diet or increase their physical activity. It's another thing to get them change the thinking that would even allow them to adopt behaviors that would help control hypertension.

This is where H-E-A-R-T can help. By encouraging you to regularly self-monitor your blood pressure, a simple and easily adopted activity that can be done in just a few seconds, you can finally bring about a change in the thinking that will help you adopt and ultimately stick with behaviors that heal hypertension and most importantly, prevent it from happening in the first place.

To lower your blood pressure and heal hypertension, I'd encourage you to do at least one of the following every day.

Avoid salty foods

The worst offenders are chips and canned soups. Look at labels. Strive for less than 2 grams of salt daily.

Drink less alcohol

If you have to drink alcohol, limit yourself to one glass of red or white wine a day and never drink on an empty stomach.

Exercise

I have yet to meet a person who didn't have at least ten to fifteen minutes a day for some sort of physical activity. Just ten minutes of walking a day can make all the difference.

Relax

Consider starting every day with ten minutes of deep breathing. During this time, think about a few goals you'd like to accomplish in the day.

Incorporate some or all of these simple activities in your daily routine and before you know it you'll "H" heal your hypertension.

CHAPTER 5

Energize: Your Heart in Motion

In this chapter you'll learn the second step for following your heart and how staying active can "E—energize your heart."

In the health and wellness field, consensus is about as hard to come by as water in the Sahara Desert. However, there is one thing that experts seem to agree on: Exercise is good for your heart. Mountains of evidence point to the countless benefits of regular physical activity and the dangers of a sedentary lifestyle. A regular exercise regimen can improve your cardiovascular health, lower blood pressure, speed up metabolism, maintain a healthy weight, reduce diabetes risk, and lower LDL cholesterol and triglycerides levels. We know this, yet research indicates that only 20 percent of us exercise regularly. Even if you count every calorie that passes your lips, you're at increased risk for cardiovascular disease if you don't exercise. Physical inactive adults are nearly twice as likely as those who are active to have coronary heart disease. This chapter clears up any confusion, spelling out the type, amount, and duration of physical activity needed to lower the risk of and ultimately prevent a cardiac event, reverse some heart disease risk factors and support the functioning of this most vital muscle.

FALLING OFF THE FITNESS BANDWAGON: KAREN'S STORY

Karen was embarrassed. Actually, horrified is more like it. For years, she'd been preaching the value of healthy living, particularly regular physical activity, to her students. Now, just days away from her thirtieth birthday, this popular high school health education teacher realized she was sixty-five pounds overweight. Teenagers are adept at sniffing out B.S. In time, the healthy lifestyle message would fall on deaf ears, especially coming from the mouth of someone who appeared to be living the opposite.

What bothered Karen even more is that she should have known better. Along with being a health education teacher, Karen was a two-sport athlete in college. It was during graduate school, Karen told me during our first consult, that things started heading south. Like most graduate students, Karen had to balance a demanding course load with research and a part-time job as a teaching assistant to undergraduates (another requirement), which left precious little time for anything else. "Exercise was the first thing to go," she said, adding that after eight years of organized athletics she didn't see anything wrong with "taking a little break." Of course, Karen never expected her "little break," would mean months of little to no physical activity. On rare days off, Karen barely found the energy to get out of bed, much less workout.

While she was abandoning exercise, she was also eating more. As a supremely conditioned high school and college athlete, Karen had always been careful about her diet, even having a doctor conduct a functional nutritional analysis of her blood to measure for levels of organic acids, fatty acids, amino acids, vitamins, minerals, and antioxidants. But those days had long passed. Things started going downhill slowly. At first it was bag of potato chips instead of an apple, or can of Coke instead of a glass of water. Before too long, fast food meals and late night pizza replaced healthy salads and lean protein, once staples of her diet. Some days she would skip meals, which played havoc with her blood sugar, and caused her to eat even more when she finally did find make time for food.

The combination of more calories and little physical activity was a double whammy for Karen. Along with weight gain, Karen's whole mood and outlook changed. Usually optimistic and upbeat, Karen turned gloomy and nihilistic. She was quick tempered, often "exploding," as she described, at her undergraduate students for no reason at all. It was easy to see why. Exercise had always been Karen's outlet for dealing with stress, not to mention the other "slings and arrows of life's misfortunes." Now that outlet was gone.

Along with the change in mood, Karen noticed changes in her physical health as well. She was tired, and often short of breath. Simply walking up a long flight of stairs left her winded, which was a great contrast to her college days when she and her teammates would spend hours running up and down the football stadium steps. She was also having intermittent chest pain, which she first attributed to normal everyday stress. But when the pain persisted, even growing in duration and frequency, she grew concerned. She visited her doctor, who performed a stress test, which came back negative. A stress test is used to detect the presence of coronary artery disease. Of course, President Clinton also had a negative stress test and soon after needed open-heart surgery, a fact not lost on Karen.

Given her concerns, Karen's doctor suggested she set up a consult with me. After conducting a full work up and reviewing the results of her stress test, I explained why she might still be experiencing symptoms. Some tests are more sensitive than others and the test her doctor performed might not have picked up anything, which could explain how President Clinton's doctors missed his advanced CAD.

To ease Karen's fear, I performed a second stress test, which this time turned up evidence of some minor blockages. I told Karen not to worry too much since this was something that could be easily treated with medication. What I told Karen I couldn't treat with medication was her behavior, which given her family background and disease-free medical history, was clearly at the root of her problems. I didn't pull any punches. "Karen you're very overweight, you're eating poorly, and you're not exercising. We dodged a bullet this time but may not get so lucky on the next go around."

At first, Karen couldn't quite believe her fall from fitness grace. But as she reflected a bit, she realized that her "fitness collapse," as she put, was a long time in the making. Karen told me she was committed to practicing what she preached and returning to a heart-healthy lifestyle.

Immediately, Karen made changes. Instead of using the elevator, she started taking the stairs to her tenth-floor apartment. During school recess, she walked a mile around the school track. Instead of leaving in her car in the teacher's only lot, she parked 5 blocks away from school and walked the rest of the way. Twice a week, she rode her bike the twenty-mile round trip to work.

Karen also made changes to her eating behavior. She cleaned out all the junk food in her house. "You can't eat what's not there," I told her. She also started packing lunch instead of going out to eat, where it's much harder to exercise portion control and monitor the ingredients. Finally, Karen did away with her habit of skipping meals, which I reminded her could lead to metabolic changes that might heighten her risk for heart disease. Habitual meal skippers have elevated fasting glucose levels and a delayed insulin response—conditions that, if they persist long term, could lead to diabetes. As a final incentive, I reminded Karen not to think of calories but to think of fingers. Every time Karen sat down to a meal or snack I told her to hold up five fingers. Any food that passed through Karen's lips should be geared toward helping her achieve the five numbers most important for reversing and preventing heart disease. Even if you just achieve one of the five numbers then you'll be on your way to achieving optimal heart health.

Before too long, the pounds came off. In just one month, Karen lost 20 pounds. After a year, she lost almost 70 pounds and was back to her ideal body weight. Soon, the daily walks turned to longer and longer jogs. A year and half after beginning her weight loss journey, Karen came in first in her age division at a town-sponsored 10K as her students, past and present, cheered her on at the finish line.

LACK OF PHYSICAL ACTIVITY: A UNIVERSAL PROBLEM

I often wonder if there's anyone who still doesn't know of all the health benefits of regular physical activity. Ask yourself: How does it feel to get out and take a walk on beautiful sunny day, go for swim, or hit the treadmill at the gym? But what seems lost is that regular physical activity is central to a heart-healthy lifestyle. Indeed, when it comes to heart health, physical inactivity is a killer. Aside from obesity, which often results from a sedentary lifestyle, physical inactivity is the biggest risk factor for cardiovascular disease. Hands down. A recent U.S. Surgeon General report supports this contention, concluding that inactive people are nearly twice as likely to develop heart disease as those who are more active.[1] And this is true even if you have no other conditions or habits that increases your risk for heart disease. Lack of physical activity also leads to more visits to the cardiologist, more hospitalizations, and more use of medicines. Physical inactivity is a recipe for disaster.

Physical activity falls under the same rubric as dieting: Something we know we should do, but don't really do. A series of research papers published in the *Lancet*, one of the world's most respected medical journals, found that worldwide physical inactivity isn't just small problem but a global pandemic. Lack of physical activity is the cause in 10 percent of premature deaths around the world each year—roughly as many as smoking.

About 5.3 million of the 57 million deaths worldwide in 2008 could be attributed to physical inactivity largely due to four major diseases: heart disease, type 2 diabetes, breast cancer and colon cancer. If physical activity could be increased by just 10 percent it might save 533,000 lives annually; if increased by 25 percent, 1.3 million lives could be saved. Taking it one step further, if we eliminated inactivity altogether, life expectancy of the world's population would rise by about 0.68 years, which is comparable to the effect of doing away with smoking or obesity.

In the *Lancet* study, scientists calculated something called a *population attributable fraction* or PAF, a measure of the contribution that physical inactivity and other risk factors make to diseases such as CAD, diabetes, and even the risk of death. The PAF told scientists how many cases of disease could theoretically be prevented if the risk factor were eliminated. In other words, what might happen if all inactive people in a population started exercising more?

After collecting data on physical inactivity and outcomes of four aforementioned diseases, as well as rates for death from all causes, they then calculated the PAFs for 123 countries. Overall, the estimates suggest that lack of exercise causes about 6 percent of heart disease, 7 percent of type 2 diabetes, and 10 percent of breast and colon cancers worldwide.

These findings should come as no surprise. In fact, I'm surprised the numbers aren't higher. Regular physical exercise is known to control and even reverse risk factors like high blood pressure, high blood sugar, and high cholesterol, and lower the subsequent risk of heart disease and diabetes. Regular physical activity keeps heart vessels healthy by inhibiting the formation of blood flow limiting atherosclerotic plaques.[2]

Current guidelines from places like the NIH's National Heart, Lung and Blood Institute recommend that adults get about 150 minutes of moderate exercise a week, which would be covered by just 30 minutes of brisk walking 5 days a week (the NHLBI recommends that kids get 60 or more minutes every day).

SURVIVAL OF THE UNFITTEST

Problem is we're not doing it. Roughly 31 percent of adults worldwide (1.5 billion people) and 80 percent of teens aren't exercising enough to meet the NHLBI standard, creating a fertile ground for chronic disease. And things are even worse here at home. We top the list as the globe's most sedentary region—with 43% of the population not exercising enough. (Rates of inactivity were lowest in southeast Asia, where many people walk or use bicycles). At least, we're no longer the fattest nation. Mexico now holds that dubious distinction with 32.8 percent of its population weighing in at obese. The U.S. comes in at a comparatively svelte 30 percent, in spite of the fact that we spend $125 billion annually on fast food alone. We have the most expensive healthcare system on the planet but we don't even make into the top 20 of the world's healthiest countries. Ugh!

According to the Centers for Disease Control and Prevention's Behavioral Risk Factor Surveillance System survey, which analyzed data collected from more than 450,000 U.S. adults ages 18 and older who were randomly called across all 50 states, just 20.6 percent of people—about 23 percent of all surveyed men and 18 percent of surveyed women—meet the total recommended amounts of exercise.

The weird part of all of this is that we're a nation obsessed with health issues. Fitness always is a hot button topic. And studies show that 15 percent of Americans have gym memberships. That's nice. However, only 8 percent of members actually use them!

The question of course is why. How did we become a nation of couch potatoes? Some of it has to do with our aging population. No one is too young or too old to work out but age does factor in. Not surprisingly, the CDC survey reported that those most likely to exercise were between the ages of 18 and 24 and account for 31 percent of all exercisers. Those least likely to engage in physical activity were ages 65 and older. This group accounted for nearly 16 percent of exercisers.

Education and physical infirmity factor in as well. More than 27 percent of the exercising adults are college graduates—the largest demographic group—while the population that never graduated from high school made up just 12 percent of exercisers. Similarly, just 13.5 of the heaviest among us (obese individuals with a BMI exceeded 30) regularly exercise. The numbers are better for overweight people (about 22 percent) but only slightly better at 26 percent for underweight/normal weight persons. Location also seemed to make a difference. The fewest adults exercise in West Virginia and Tennessee (less than 13 percent of exercisers for each), and the most adults exercise in Colorado (more than 27 percent of exercisers).

Modern conveniences no doubt contributed to the problem. In this country, fewer than 4 percent of people walk to work and an even smaller number—2 percent—bike to the office. Compare that to about 20 percent of walkers in China, Germany, and Sweden, and the more than 20 percent who bike to the job in countries like China, Denmark, and the Netherlands. And we sit, a lot. Meals, the office, in front of the computer, watching TV—seems like we're on our butts more than we are on our feet. And though lack of physical activity is a known risk factor for heart disease, it doesn't warrant the same attention as other risk factors like hypertension, high blood sugar, and elevated cholesterol.

THE COUCH POTATO GENE

Sometimes when I'm working late in my home office, I'll take a break to look at my daughters' pet hamster. There's something very soothing about just watching her move about and explore the elaborate little habitat my girls have constructed for her. Hamsters are crepuscular and much to my children's dismay, most active after they call it a day. Most nights, she spends hours on her running wheel. I can't imagine her going a night without it. She just loves to run and move about. I suspect its encoded into her DNA, though I don't know if anyone has yet discovered a hamster exercise gene. I wonder what her behavior says about us. Like the little hamster, are we hard wired to move, to exercise? Or, given our druthers, would we make a beeline for the nearest couch, remote in one hand, chips in the other? Does the motivation to exercise—or not—have a genetic component?

It's an interesting question. In a study out of the University of Missouri, researchers inbred two very distinct groups of rats: one of which *felt* the need to move and the other which eschewed any form of exercise, preferring instead to lay down until the *feeling* passed. Then the scientists closely scrutinized and compared the animals' bodies, brains and DNA.

Earlier studies comparing physical activity patterns among family members, found that close relations—twins as an example—have similar exercise habits, exercising about as much or as little as their closest relatives, even if they grew up in different environments. This is similar to the twin studies done in Europe that looked at the role of DNA in predicting the risk for drug addiction.

It seems hard to gauge whether the motivation to exercise is programmed into our genes or whether environmental influences such as upbringing and parenting style weigh more heavily in the decision. What the scientists found is that the gym rats spontaneously exercised ten times more than their couch potato compadres.

The question is why did they exercise more. Writing in an article in the *New York Times,* the seasoned health journalist Gretchen Reynolds observed that "two elements are especially likely to influence whether we...habitually exercise or not." Physique, she points out, is one, which makes complete sense since overweight and obese people or animals that may be ill or have other impediments to exercises will gravitate toward the nearest place to sit.

But the researchers were surprised to find that body type didn't factor much at all. Differences in physique didn't account for differences in exercise behavior. This led the researchers to examine the other primary determinant of exercise behavior: Our brains. How closely rats' emotions echo our own, if at all, is hard to know. The exercising rats enjoyed their treadmill time, while the couch potatoes studiously avoided it.

This is the point where DNA factored in, as scientists found dozens of genes that differed between the two groups, specifically those in the ventral midbrain, the ventral tegmental area, or VTA, that are involved in reward processing and the motivation to do things because they're fun or pleasurable. The VTA is the same area of the brain that goes into hyper drive when exposed to drugs of abuse. To run or not to run was being driven in part by the same mechanisms the drive us to addiction.

What does this mean for us? Could there really a gene that motivates us to run marathons and another gene that predisposes us to become glued to the remote control? Maybe. But to revisit the line I used earlier from celebrity diet doctor Stephen Gullo, PhD, "Genes impel, they don't compel." Biology isn't destiny. You can't fall back on your genes as an excuse for why you're surgically attached to the couch. When it comes to exercise, maladaptive behavior really is the number one risk factor. Even if you'd prefer to languish in bed than head out for a brisk jog, unless you're physically disabled, the decision to exercise is firmly under your control.

EXERCISE AND YOUR HEART

The heart is a muscle, nothing more, nothing less. Like all muscles, it's got an ego. It wants to do good. And it will look better and work more efficiently with regular physical activity. Exercise makes the heart stronger, allowing it to pump more blood through our bodies with less effort. Legendary tennis player Bjorn Borg, whose physical conditioning was unrivalled during his playing days, reportedly had one of the lowest resting heart rates of any professional athlete—an astonishing thirty-eight beats per minute. In all likelihood, his resting heart was closer to fifty but the story points out that the resting heart rate of those who exercise is also slower, because less effort is needed to pump blood.

Exercise has a number of effects that benefit the heart and circulatory system, including improving cholesterol and fat levels, reducing inflammation in the arteries, helping weight loss programs, and helping to keep blood vessels flexible and open.

Even patients with heart failure, a condition where the heart doesn't pump blood around the body efficiently, can benefit from exercise. Historically, heart failure patients have been discouraged from exercising. Those were the old days. Now exercise performed under medical supervision is proving helpful for select patients with stable (no decompensation) heart failure. In particular, progressive resistance has been shown to improve arterial blood flow

People who maintain an active lifestyle have a 45 percent lower risk of developing heart disease than do sedentary people. Guidelines aside, it's still an open question as to how much exercise is needed to benefit the heart. What's known, however, are the effects of exercise on the following risk factors.

HIGH CHOLESTEROL (CAD)

Beneficial changes in cholesterol and lipid levels, including lower LDL levels, occur even when people performed low amounts of moderate- or high-intensity exercise, such as walking or jogging twelve miles a week. However, more intense exercise is required to significantly change cholesterol levels, notably increasing HDL ("good" cholesterol). An example of this kind of intense program would be jogging about twenty miles a week. Benefits occur even with very modest weight loss, suggesting that overweight people who have trouble losing pounds can still achieve considerable heart benefits by exercising.

Some studies suggest that for the greatest heart protection, it is not the duration of a single exercise session that counts but the total weekly amount of energy expended.

Resistance (weight) training has also been associated with heart protection. It may offer a complementary benefit to aerobics. If you have heart disease or risk factors for heart disease, check with your doctor before starting resistance training.

BLOOD PRESSURE (HYPERTENSION)

"Exercise remains a cornerstone therapy for the primary prevention, treatment, and control of [high blood pressure]," declares *Medicine & Science in Sports & Exercise*, the official journal of the American College of Sports Medicine. Physically inactive people have a 35 percent greater risk of developing high blood pressure than physically active people. How wonderful is exercise for hypertension? *High blood pressure can be reduced for as many as twenty-two hours following a single exercise session!* A reduction in blood pressure following a single exercise session is a phenomenon known as post-exercise hypotension (PEH).

Aerobic activities like brisk walking, jogging, cycling, or swimming are best. These activities should be performed a minimum of three days per week for thirty to sixty minutes, but could be done daily. The intensity should be in the moderate range, with heart rates representing 40 to 70 percent of heart rate reserve. Resistance training activities should be done two times per week, with an emphasis on lower weight but higher repetitions (eight to twelve per set).

Always remember the "H" in H-E-A-R-T and have your blood pressure checked on a regular basis to make sure your numbers are

BLOOD PRESSURE: DOES EXERCISE ALWAYS MAKE A DIFFERENCE?

You'd be hard pressed to find a cardiologist who didn't think exercise was helpful for reducing, controlling, and even preventing high blood pressure. Regular exercise over the course of a few months can lead to a reduction in both systolic and diastolic blood pressure readings. However, there's a group that seem impervious to the blood pressure-lowering effects of exercise.

Indeed, moderate exercise may not be enough to control mild hypertension in people over age 55, according to the findings of a four-year study by Johns Hopkins University researchers. These findings bring scrutiny to the efficacy of the American College of Sports Medicine' guidelines on exercise for lowering blood pressure in older people.

Current guidelines from the American College of Sports Medicine recommend thirty- to forty-five-minute periods of combined aerobic exercise and moderate weightlifting, three to five times per week, with a corresponding reduction of eight millimeters to ten millimeters of mercury (mm/Hg).

Exercise physiologist Kerry J. Stewart, Ed.D., professor of medicine and director of clinical and research exercise physiology programs at The Johns Hopkins University School of Medicine and its Heart Institute, and lead author of the four-year long study, told the online magazine *Science Daily,* "Exercise is highly recommended for reducing blood pressure and is part of prevention and treatment programs for an estimated 90 percent of adults in the United States who eventually develop hypertension. But current exercise guidelines were based on studies that had several limitations, including that they were not tested in older adults."

Earlier studies looked at younger people, for whom hypertension has different characteristics and causes than are seen in older people. High cardiac output, where the heart beats faster than it has to both at rest and during exercise, is most often the cause of hypertension in younger

(continues)

(continued)

(under fifty-five) adults. Hypertension in mature adults is a consequence of *arterial stiffening* where the walls of the large arteries that carry blood throughout the body become less elastic or flexible. This condition triggers a rise in blood pressure.

Over a six-month period, The SHAPE (Senior Hypertension and Physical Exercise) study tracked the blood pressure of 104 men and women between the ages fifty-five to seventy-five. Half were given a moderate exercise program while the rest maintained their usual physical routine and diet.

At the beginning of the study, most participants had systolic hypertension, when the systolic blood pressure is high and the diastolic blood pressure is normal. Systolic hypertension is more common in people over age fifty-five.

At the conclusion of the study, exercisers showed significant improvements in overall fitness and body composition—increased lean muscle mass and reduced fat, especially abdominal fat. But the participants didn't fare as well with blood pressure, with the special exercise group lowering systolic blood pressure by 5.3 mm/Hg and the non-exercise group by 4.5 mm/Hg, which isn't considered statistically significant. Arterial stiffness also didn't improve in either group (diastolic reductions were much greater for exercisers).

The researchers found that people most likely to decrease both systolic and diastolic blood pressure also were those who lost the most body fat, particularly abdominal fat, and gained the most muscle.

Additional data show that both high intensity and low intensity training lowered blood pressure during exercise and when checked in the doctor's office. Only high intensity training had effects on body fat, weight and cholesterol levels. So in general I tell my patients that any exercise, when part of your daily routine, is good for your heart. Sometimes individualized exercise regimens need to be created for patients with known cardiovascular conditions.

within an ideal range. Some people may require medication, but I've found that lifestyle modifications, including the foods in the *5 For 1 Diet* do the trick. If exercise alone doesn't lower high blood pressure, it can help with weight control, reduce cholesterol, and stabilize blood sugar.

Anyone with existing high blood pressure should discuss an exercise program with their doctor. Before starting to exercise, people with moderate-to-severe high blood pressure should lower their blood pressure, and be able to control it with medications. Everyone, especially people with high blood pressure, should breathe as normally as possible through each exercise. Holding the breath increases blood pressure.

ELEVATED BLOOD GLUCOSE

If you've ever gone for a long run on a warm humid day then you'll know that maintaining blood sugar during exercise can be challenging. Even in healthy people, hypoglycemia always is a risk during exercise. It follows that exercise poses a great challenge for diabetics, especially for those who take insulin.

Still, regular exercise is critical and it is known to lower blood sugar levels. Muscles use glucose as fuel, so in theory any type of activity can reduce blood sugar levels. Exercise also helps the body use insulin more efficiently, which in turn, helps the body use more glucose.

And you don't even need to work out for hours, as recent research suggests that just seventy-five minutes of high intensity exercise time a week could lower blood sugar levels for twenty-four hours after exercise, and help prevent post-meal blood sugar spikes in people with type 2 diabetes.

In our time-pressed society, shorter workouts seem to be the rage, and I agree that if you only have ten minutes to spare it's better than nothing. But to get all of the benefits of exercise, I suggest you follow the current recommendations from the American Diabetes

Association of at least 150 minutes of moderate to vigorous exercise each week, or thirty minutes a day, five days a week. Remember the more you work out, the more your muscles will demand glucose, their primary food source.

Need more proof? It's believed that pre-meal exercise helps regulate blood sugar levels almost as well as Metformin and Pioglitazone, two common glucose-lowering medications. How? It may be that exercising on an empty stomach, particularly first thing in the morning after eight to twelve hours of fasting, might empty out the liver's supply of whatever glycogen—the body's sugar source—prompting a signal the brain to lower its demand for sugar. This could be welcome to diabetics, allowing them to substitute medication for a vigorous morning workout.[2]

WEIGHT CONTROL

"How much exercise do I need to keep my weight down Dr. Kennedy?" A day doesn't go by when I'm not asked that very question. But there's no hard and fast rule as to how much activity you will need to maintain a healthy a weight. In fact, exercise's contribution to weight loss isn't all it's cracked up to be. By no means do I mean to imply that you shouldn't exercise, particularly if you're overweight. I exercise almost every day. I don't view it any differently than brushing my teeth.

But exercise, it turns out, is no weight-loss panacea. All physical activity burns calories. That's no great scientific revelation. Given that reality, exercise should play a critical role in weight loss. The problem is that people use exercise as a license to gorge, thinking the hour or so spent at the gym a few times a week is will allow them to eat to their heart's content. You burn a pound of fat whenever you burn 3500 calories more than you consume. Think about how much exercise you'd need to shed just 10 pounds without changing your diet. To lose just 10 pounds you'd have to create a 35,000-calorie deficit. That's a lot of hours on the treadmill.

Few people grasp how difficult it is to exercise enough to lose weight. Unless you're a professional athlete, whose job it is to work-out, you're not going to burn enough calories alone to lose weight. Depending on your weight, even a vigorous 45-minute spin class wouldn't burn up more than 500 calories, which you could easily wipeout with a post workout bran muffin and 16-oz latte.

While exercise doesn't make us thin, its role in weight mainte-nance, or weight control, is paramount. A *Journal of the American Medical Association* study that followed the exercise habits of 34,000 women concluded that an hour a day of moderate (3 mph walking) exercising was need to maintain weight. This research supports Na-tional Weight Control Registry findings that 90 percent of people who successfully lose weight and kept it off exercise for 60 minutes a day on average.

The general consensus about exercise is increase intensity and shorten the time, a formula that seems to increase the health bene-fits and ramp up fat burning. I tell patients to exercise for H-E-A-R-T but don't expect a daily three-mile walk with friends to leave you with sculpted six-pack abs, bulging biceps, or a tightly toned tush, particularly if you don't change your way of eating.

FOODS TO FUEL WORKOUTS

Mountain climbing or mall walking...an hour of tennis or vigorous game of shuffle board—no matter how you decide to burn some calories, you need some fuel in the tank otherwise you're in store for a very short ride. Below is a list of my nine foods that will keep your heart humming before, during and after a workout.

Low Fat Dairy—Low-fat dairy foods are rich in vitamin D, calcium, and other important minerals to help preserve fat-burning muscle mass. This makes yogurt and cheese ideal pre-workout snacks.

(continues)

(continued)

Bananas—Grab a banana before a sweat session for a healthy hit of carbs. The yellow fruit is also high in potassium, a mineral that helps keep cells hydrated.

Oatmeal—Don't want to crash and burn mid-workout? Try a cup of whole-grain oatmeal. It's packed with heart-healthy fiber to prevent blood sugar spikes.

Quinoa—Quinoa is a super grain that's high in protein and complex carbs. It contains tons of iron, fiber, and calcium to aid muscle contraction, plus electrolytes for good hydration.

Walnuts—Grab a handful of these nuts before you work out: Studies show their omega 3s may prevent post-workout binges that cancel out the calories you burn. They're loaded with minerals to aid metabolism too.

Mandarin Oranges—This sweet treat hydrates a workout with energy-fueling carbs and vitamin C. Studies suggest the sunshine vitamin boosts a workout's fat-burning potential.

Apples & Peanut Butter—Munch on this dynamic duo before you sweat to pump up stamina and prevent blood sugar spikes. After a workout, they replenish energy stores without bogging down digestion.

Scrambled Eggs—This quick and easy post-workout meal is low in calories and high in muscle-replenishing proteins. Toss in a generous amount of veggies to add fiber and antioxidants.

Salmon—Salmon is a tasty and satisfying way to replenish the body after a workout. A lean protein, this oily fish contains hormonal-balancing omega 3s and magnesium to help you stay lean and toned.

STARTING OUT

If you have heart disease, any of the known risk factors for developing heart disease, or if you're sedentary but otherwise perfectly healthy, I suggest you consult with your healthcare provider before starting an exercise program. If you're at risk, you need to be aware of the symptoms that could spell trouble (see the box).

IS FAT THE NEW FIT?

"I'm in shape," a friend of mine repeatedly quips at the gym. "Round is a shape."

It's an old joke, but there may be some truth to it. Is it possible to be both overweight, obese even, and healthy?

You wouldn't think so given that obesity is linked to dozens of chronic health conditions. However, there seems to a miraculous a sub-set of obese people who seem to be protected from obesity-related metabolic complications.

Blood pressure, triglycerides, cholesterol, and high fasting glucose levels determine optimal metabolic health. But people who are obese and healthy, meaning they don't have any of the listed risk factors have what scientists now refer to as "uncomplicated obesity" or "metabolically benign obesity," meaning their obesity has no obvious adverse health effects.

Metabolically healthy but also obese people have a significantly lower risk of dying than their metabolically unhealthy peers. Taking it one step further, metabolically healthy and obese people are in just as good a shape as healthy normal weight folks.

How is that possible?

There is some evidence that cardiorespiratory fitness make us healthier irrespective of our weight. Does this mean that we should all go out and chow down on cheeseburgers, fries and milkshakes? No, not exactly.

Being fat is still the biggest risk factor in my estimation for CAD. We see insulin resistance, as an example, far more often in overweight people. Also, duration of obesity, as we've discussed throughout the book, also factors into metabolic risk.

Still, there is little doubt as to the hearth healthy benefits of regular exercise, whether you're fit or fat.[3]

Before recommending specific exercises to patients, I have them fill out a simple questionnaire.

Has any doctor previously recommended medically supervised activity because of a heart condition?
Does physical activity bring on chest pain?
Has chest pain occurred during the previous month?
Do you have a history of fainting or dizziness?
Do bone or joint pain intensify during or after exercise?
Are you taking medication for heart disease or any of the known risk factors?
Do you have a medical condition that could keep you from exercising or put you at increased risk?
If you answered "yes" to any of these questions, I'd strongly encourage you to get a full medical evaluation before exercising.

I also frequently recommend a *stress test, especially for non-exercisers,* to help determine the risk for any problems resulting from exercise.

IS THE ROAD TO HELL PAVED WITH GOOD INTENTIONS?

Albeit small, a percentage of heart attacks occur after heavy physical exercise and mostly in people who are already at high risk for a coronary event. Are you one of those people? You need to find out. In general, the following people should avoid intense exercise or begin only with careful monitoring by a healthcare professional.

- If you have an underlying medical condition such as uncontrolled diabetes, seizures, high blood pressure, heart failure, unstable angina, significant aortic valve disease, or aortic aneurysm. People with moderate-to-severe hypertension (systolic blood pressure over 160 mm Hg or diastolic pressure over 100 mm Hg) should have

(continues)

(continued)

  their blood pressure brought down to the normal range before beginning a vigorous exercise program.

- If you've spent the better part of your life glued to your La-Z Boy chair, particularly if you're older (over age 55). Episodes of exercise-related sudden death in young people are rare. Fainting precedes some, which is due to a sudden and severe drop in blood pressure. Fainting or syncope is even common in professional and accomplished amateur athletes often the result of dehydration or post performance hypoglycemia, but only considered dangerous for those with existing heart conditions.

- There's some debate as to whether people with genetic or congenital heart disorders should avoid intensive competitive sports. Marfan syndrome, a genetic disorder of the body's connective tissue of which the most serious symptoms involve the heart and cardiovascular system, is just such a condition and has claimed the lives of several high profile professional athletes, including former U.S. volleyball star Flo Hyman. Marfan sufferers have to avoid all contact sports due to an increased risk of aortic rupture. The National Marfan Foundation has a complete list of guidelines for physical activity on its website. Anabolic steroids and ephedra-based products have been linked to numerous incidents of stroke, heart attack, and even death. Ephedra, as an example, is a vasoconstrictor, meaning it narrows blood vessels and could increase the risk of a coronary event. Still, even in high-risk individuals, some form of carefully monitored exercise is most often beneficial. In my experience, age and a sedentary lifestyle are the biggest risk factors for problems

- If you're at risk, you may want to avoid intense physical activity, especially if you're over age 55. Shoveling, running, race-walking, singles tennis, weight lifting, spinning, and heavy gardening fit the "intense" workout bill. Even in healthy people, these workouts stress the heart, raise blood pressure for brief periods, and

(continues)

(continued)

may cause arterial spasms. Certain competitive sports, such as basketball, soccer, mixed martial arts, boxing, and ice hockey, which couple intense physical activity with aggressive emotions, are more likely to trigger a heart attack or even cardiac arrest than other forms of exercise. Though it's worth pointing out that participants in these sports tend to be well conditioned and have had an extensive medical workup prior to competing.

No matter what your sport or activity level, I encourage you to listen for warning signs. It's been estimated that 40% of young men who die suddenly during exercise previously experienced, and ignored, warning signs of heart disease.[4] In addition to avoiding risky activities, the best preventive tactic is simply to listen to the body and seek medical help at the first sign of symptoms during or following exercise. These symptoms include the following:

- Irregular heartbeat
- Shortness of breath
- Chest pain

ENERGIZING FOR A HEALTHY H-E-A-R-T

You know the Nike spot, "Just do it."

Research points out that simply getting off your duff will improve your numbers, especially blood cholesterol and triglycerides, blood sugar and hypertension. And except in rare instances, physical disability is no excuse. Just becoming slightly more active—using stairs instead of the elevator as an example—or paying more attention to your ambient environment—a study found that improving lighting can boost activity levels by as much as 50 percent—can do wonders.

CHAPTER 6

Body Mass Index: Apples, Pears, and Your Heart

In this chapter you'll learn the third step of following your heart by "A—Acting on Fat."

You've probably heard the news. A major study of 220,000 people published in the prestigious Lancet Medical Journal has challenged the long-held idea that obese people who carry their extra weight mainly around the middle — those with an "apple" shape — are at greater risk for heart disease than "pears," or those whose fat tends to cluster on their thighs and buttocks. When it comes to cardiovascular disease, said the study, it's not your shape but being overweight or obese that is a primary risk factor for cardiovascular disease. Although there is data showing the opposite, that body shape is predictive of heart disease, it's a cold heart fact that those that eat more apples and pears (as long as it's not a crate at a time) are at lower risk for developing cardiovascular disease. Simply, if you're overweight, you're at increased risk, no matter where you carry your weight. The good news is that you can reduce your risk of cardiovascular disease by maintaining a healthy weight no matter what your shape. What's your waist size? What's your shape? Where does your body collect fat? What are your body mass index and waist-to-hip ratio? And what can you do today to achieve ideal numbers? This chapter offers answers to these critical questions, giving us a better understanding our personal risk of cardiovascular disease, and the actions and steps needed to achieve and maintain optimal heart health.

PREACHING WHAT HE SHOULD BE PRACTICING: MIKE'S STORY

Around campus, Mike was simply "the man." Unlike his less gifted medical school classmates, Mike was blessed with a photographic memory and an uncanny ability to absorb complex information "like a sponge," as one of our professors put it. I met Mike during our first year at Dartmouth Medical School (now the Geisel School of Medicine). Most of us were just in bewildered awe of Mike.

Predictably, Mike would go on to graduate at the top of our class, which he followed up with one of the most sought after residencies in internal medicine at Harvard's famed Brigham & Women's Hospital. Within two years, Mike was promoted to chief resident. After completing his residency, Mike became one of the hospital's most respected attending physicians, and a man admired greatly by colleagues, medical students and patients alike. Mike was an astute clinician whose phenomenal training, and easy way with people paved the way for him to open a thriving practice.

On the home front, Mike's beautiful wife had just given birth to their first child, a girl. Everything was going great for Mike, except for one small detail—there was something missing. He'd confide to friends that though he should be "the happiest guy in the world," he was restless and bored. "I don't know what it is," he told me over dinner one night. Truth is, Mike was finding it hard to balance the demands of a thriving medical practice with his desire spend more time with his young family. He was working sixteen-hour days, leaving his wife to complain that he spends "more time with his patients than he does with his family." Something had to give.

After much soul searching, Mike decided to close his outpatient clinic, electing to become a full time hospitalist (physicians who care for you while you are hospitalized). Although this new schedule allowed Mike to be around home more during the day, he paid for it at night, where on any given night he could be paged twenty times and always between 2 and 6 AM, which made sleep difficult. This new schedule, while requiring fewer hours, placed even heavier physical and emotional demands on Mike. He was habitually exhausted, which left him cranky and irritable. "I did this to make things easier, but now I feel worse than I did when I was cranking out sixteen hour days," he told me.

To keep pace, Mike started pounding energy drinks, which contain four to five times more caffeine per serving than an eight-ounce cup of coffee and depending on the brand, upwards of 200 calories per serving. Normally careful about his diet, Mike found his new schedule barely allowed him time to eat, much less sit down to a meal. He'd often "grab and go," picking up whatever was in arm's reach as he was running out the door to see a patient. Or, he'd stop for a donut and an energy drink on the way to the hospital. He needed something to get the juices flowing at 2 AM.

After returning home from the hospital early one morning, Mike was thrilled to find his daughter, who'd just turned one, playing happily in her jump-a-roo. As he bent over to pick her up, a remarkable thing happened: the button on his trousers popped. He'd noticed that some of his pants hadn't been fitting right, but he attributed that to normal laundry shrinkage. But just to be just sure, Mike jumped on the scale. He was shocked. In just nine months, Mike's had ballooned from 160 to 210. That's a lot of extra weight to carry on a 5'9" frame. Even worse, his waist size had mushroomed from a healthy 32 to 40. As a physician, Mike knew about the risks of carrying excess fat around the mid-section. But as a self-professed "guy who gets things done," he was confident that he'd take the weight off in record time. "Piece of cake," Mike told his wife.

After a particularly stressful night at the hospital, Mike felt a strong sudden pain in his chest, just as he was calling in a prescription for a patient. He'd never experienced anything like this. Mike knew all the numbers about heart attacks. He didn't want to become another statistic. Concerned, he called 911. Paramedics arrived soon after and took Mike to the hospital.

The term "heart pain" is misleading since it's doesn't always herald a heart attack and isn't always in the chest. For that reason, I prefer the Latin term *angina pectoris* or "sensation in the chest," to describe chest pain. This is not just a vocabulary lesson; it's a life lesson. People die because they don't realize that significance of chest pain, opting to ignore obvious symptoms and risk a heart attack.

Mike's numbers came back negative for any cardiovascular problems. And his chest pain, which he described to the attending physician—and one of his closest friends—as sharp and brief that worsened when he moved too much, was not from the heart but from a severely strained muscle in his chest.

Of greater concern to Mike's colleague and friend was the noticeable weight gain. "Mike, no offense, but how did you gain so much weight?" That was all Mike needed to hear. It was one thing for his wife to nag him about a few extra pounds but it was another matter altogether to hear a genuine expression of concern from a fellow physician. As someone who treated hundreds of patients struggling with weight issues, Mike knew the devastating effect that just a few extra pounds could cause. That night, Mike calculated his BMI, which was a shocking 30.4, putting him right over the edge into the "obese" category. Even worse, his waist to hip ratio was a shocking +1.0, putting him at risk for a host of illnesses including coronary heart disease, diabetes and hypertension. Your health isn't solely affected by your weight or even how much body fat you have, but also where that fat is disturbed on your body. Unfortunately for Mike, most of the weight had collected around his waist. He had developed an apple shaped body, which is far more common in men than women (men tend to gain weight around the middle; women gain in their hips, thighs and buttocks).

Though many studies indicate that genes determine our body shape and weight, Mike was clearly in a prison of his own making. In fact, most of his biological family was thin. Mike's environment and personal choices were having the greatest impact on his weight. Our genes have been around for millions of years but the overweight and obesity epidemic is a twenty-first century phenomenon.

A few days after his "health scare," Mike called me up. He seemed more embarrassed than concerned about what had happened. "I don't know how I let this happen, John. I'm a physician for heaven's sake." I told Mike not to stress too much and that physicians, despite handing out medical advice for a living, don't always practice what they preach. I don't like taking medicine, even aspirin, unless it's absolutely necessary. I reminded Mike that his recent weight gain was no "fat sentence," and that with a little creative strategy, which included an abrupt end to his six-a-day energy drink habit, he'd be back to his normal weight in no time.

To borrow a line from Dr. Stephen Gullo, bestselling author of *Thin Tastes Better* and the *Thin Commandments Diet* and architect of the food strategy approach to weight control: "Genes impel, they don't compel." At the end of the day, with the right strategies you're in the driver's seat of your own life. Genes and environment notwithstanding, you won't gain extra weight if you're expending more calories than you're taking in. Even if you were born a pear or apple you can be the fittest fruit possible.

THE SKINNY ON BMI

Most of us don't need a scientific formula to know if we are fat. All we have to do is look in the mirror, struggle to button our pants, or gaze longingly at the thin and handsome face in our senior year-book. But for the majority of people, the only number that really matters is the number on the bathroom scale (though as we'll see later, weight alone can be a misleading indication of overall health).

Many of us know the weight we'd like to be. But that often enters the realm of fantasy. What's more important is a weight we can really expect to maintain. Therein lies the problem. How do we know what constitutes a "healthy weight?" A recent Google search of the term turned up 178 million hits! Getting a straightforward answer can seem all but impossible. A 6-foot, 260-pound Division I college football player would have a BMI of 33.9, making him "medically obese." But few Division I athletes I'm aware of are obese, much less overweight. In all likelihood, it's muscle or lean body mass, which weighs more than fat, that accounts for the high BMI. In fact, if this same player were to quit football and stop working out his BMI would probably drop, though it would be hard to argue that he was "fitter" after quitting.

Because BMI only measures weight and height, there's no way it can assess the difference between lean mass and fat, a critical variable in assessing disease risk. A 2008 study that looked at more than 13,000 people found that 21 percent of men and 31 percent of women met the BMI criteria for obesity (BMI > 30). However, after measuring body fat percentage, which BMI doesn't do, obesity was found in 50% of men and 62% of women.

Clearly, weight alone is a misleading way of assessing the risk of heart disease. If two women walk into my office—both 160 pounds—I can't simply use weight to assess their health risk. If one woman is 5'11" and the other 5'2", it doesn't take a genius to realize that the taller woman—with a BMI of 22.3—has a healthy weight but the 5'2" woman—BMI 29.3—is overweight and almost obese. It's not fair—life seldom is. But exceptions aside, the shorter person cannot carry the same weight on a smaller frame. Most of the time, whether you're a man or woman, carrying around 160 pounds on a

CALCULATING YOUR BMI

To my mind, BMI is a description of a person's body size based on his or her height and weight. But how to you calculate your BMI? For most of my patients, I recommend they use the BMI calculator provided by the National Center for Chronic Disease Prevention and Health Promotion (http://www.cdc.gov/healthyweight/assessing/bmi/). They provide BMI calculators for both adults and children. Simply enter your height and weight and press the "calculate" button and you'll instantly have your BMI. If you don't have a computer, or the latest mobile phone, you can calculate your own BMI using the following formula.

$$\text{BMI} = [(\text{weight in pounds}) \div (\text{height inches})^2] \times 703$$

The BMI calculation is the same for men and women, which is part of its drawback. After figuring out your BMI, follow the chart below (courtesy of the National Heart, Lung and Blood Institute) to see how you rate.

Height	21	22	23	24	25	26	27	28	29	30	31
4'10"	100	105	110	115	119	124	129	134	138	143	148
5'0"	107	112	118	123	128	133	138	143	148	153	158
5'1"	111	116	122	127	132	137	143	148	153	158	164
5'3"	118	124	130	135	141	146	152	158	163	169	175
5'5"	126	132	138	144	150	156	162	168	174	180	186
5'7"	134	140	146	153	159	166	172	178	185	191	198
5'9"	142	149	155	162	169	176	182	189	196	203	209
5'11"	150	157	165	172	179	186	193	200	208	215	222
6'1"	159	166	174	182	189	197	204	212	219	227	235
6'3"	168	176	184	192	200	208	216	224	232	240	248

BMI is generally divided into four categories. A score of 19–24 is normal; 25–29 is overweight; 30–39 is obese; and over 40 extreme or morbid obesity. There are other categories as well, including underweight (BMI 17–19) and anorexic (under 17) and even super obese (over 50). Again, these numbers may be misleading since a perfectly fit and healthy ballerina measuring 5'5" and 110 pounds would be viewed as "underweight." The numbers are a little easier to make sense of in the obese/super obese category since I've never encountered anyone with a BMI over 40, much less 50, that I'd term "healthy," no matter how tall or fit they might be.

5'2" frame makes you fat. The relationship between height and weight can't be overestimated.

I understand the frustration many people have with the BMI system. It's inherently flawed. I wouldn't argue otherwise. There's little wiggle room before you're assigned a category. For instance, a 5'2" person who weighs 131 pounds has a BMI of 24. If this person gains just five pounds, then her BMI increases to 25—which puts her into the overweight zone. At the opposite end of the spectrum, a 5'2" person can weigh as little as 104 pounds before falling into the underweight category (BMI < 19). These little "cutoff numbers" don't seem fair. What if our 5'2" woman started bodybuilding, CrossFit training, or any other form of exercise that rapidly builds muscle? By BMI standards, if she added five pounds she'd cross into the "overweight" category, even though that weight gain may have come from muscle, not fat. The same problems apply to any statistical measurement. Blood pressure is an obvious example. Though the definition of these transition points is based on sound scientific data, who's to say where normal blood pressure ends and high blood pressure begins? And when it comes to body weight, the definition does seem a little arbitrary.

BMI also doesn't take into account the proportions of muscle, bone, and fat. I already explained the potential disconnect in weight gain from fat and weight gain from muscle. As might be expected, the BMI is not too helpful in these situations. BMI would be useless for looking at a muscle bound, 5'8" 190-pound tailback with 6 percent body fat. No one would dare call him "fat," but his BMI of 29.9 puts him firmly in the "overweight" category.

Fat distribution also is something beyond the scope of the BMI. A 5'10" 170-pound man is at the far end of the "normal" weight range. But what if that man happens to carry most of that weight in his abdomen? He's an apple shape and though he's technically within the normal weight category, he's also at risk for a host of diseases associated with the proverbial potbelly. Another 5'10" 170-pound

---

CALCULATING YOUR WAIST-TO-HIP RATIO

Waist circumference is measured by wrapping a flexible measuring tape around your natural (unclothed) waist (in between the lowest rib and the top of the hip bone), the belly button, or at the narrowest point of the midsection. When measuring, keep the tape parallel to the floor.

Hip circumference is measured by wrapping a flexible tape around the hips at the widest diameter of the buttocks. Keep the tape parallel to the floor.

To calculate your waist to hip ratio, divide your waist circumference by your hip circumference.

---

man who carries his weight in his hips and thighs—pear-shaped—would have fewer health risks.

It's not fair because the BMI doesn't accurately assess excessive body fat. There are other ways to describe body weight distribution, and there are more accurate methods for measuring body fat. Currently the BMI does not work such concepts into its formula. Remember this: the BMI is an example of scientists trying to impose order on a human characteristic. Such behavior can create an artificial situation, which can lead to inaccuracies.

Despite these drawbacks, BMI is part of the healthy lifestyle zeitgeist. And since it's an easy thing to calculate, and readily accessible with a computer or mobile device, it's an important part of any discussion of weight and cardiovascular health. BMI provides a common language for doctors, researchers, and patients to discuss weight issues. The BMI is not the best gauge of body fat, but it's what we have right now. That's why I use the BMI in my practice every day, which along with hip-to-waist ratio is good at predicting the risk of heart disease and even a fatal cardiac event.

The first major study to connect the dots between BMI, waist size, and heart disease was published in the *European Journal of*

Cardiovascular Prevention and Rehabilitation (now called the *European Journal of Preventive Cardiology*). In the study, which looked at 20,000 men and women between the ages 20–65, 50 percent of fatal, and 25 percent of non-fatal heart disease in overweight and obese people could be explained by BMI. Though other studies have tied body mass index to heart disease, the uniqueness of this particular study was that it did not rely upon self-reported data (BMI alone). Instead, anthropometric (body research) measurements were used. When BMI and waist size were adjusted for age, and correlated to cause-of-death stats and hospital records, people who were classified as overweight or obese (based on BMI and waist size), 53 percent of the fatal heart disease, and 25–30 percent of the non-fatal heart disease.[1]

As we've discussed throughout this book, abdominal fat is insidious because it's a deep, or more properly termed "visceral" fat that surrounds the internal organs. Abdominal fat promotes insulin resistance and unhealthy cholesterol numbers, and likely contributes to inflammation.

THE OBESITY PARADOX: FACT OR FICTION

Obesity increases a person's risk of heart disease. That's no great shock. But things might not be as clear as we once thought. It could be that a high body mass index is associated with a *lower* risk of dying from heart disease and other chronic illnesses—a mysterious phenomenon known as the "obesity paradox."

The paradox can be explained by one simple fact: BMI is a very flawed measure of heart risk. On the other hand, waist size is a far more accurate way to gauge the risk of suffering a cardiac event, the study found. Patients with large waist size—more than 35 inches for women and 40 inches for men—are 70 percent more likely to die during the

(continues)

(continued)

study period than those with smaller waists. Predictably, a combination of a large waist and a high BMI upped the risk of death significantly. What seems to matter more than anything is the distribution of fat.

Given the study findings, what are we to make of BMI as a tool for assessing the risk of a coronary event? Indeed, there are serious problems with BMI as a measuring tool. For one, BMI doesn't measure body shape—apple or pear—or fat distribution. BMI also doesn't distinguish between fat and muscle (muscle weighs more than fat). So a perfectly fit and healthy NFL defensive lineman could very well have a high BMI. Heart patients who lead a sedentary lifestyle may see a drop in BMI if they lose muscle mass, while heart-disease patients who become more active may actually put on weight via lean muscle and raise their BMI.

The findings also add fuel to the debate surrounding body type and the risk of developing heart disease. Several studies have suggested that people with an apple-shaped body who accumulate fat in their belly are more likely to develop heart disease than their pear-shaped counterparts. A study from the Mayo clinic found that central obesity was a more accurate predictor of death than high BMI. Using data collected from five separate studies of 15,547 participants with CAD in five studies on three continents, researchers looked at mortality risk based on measurement of both body mass index (BMI) and central obesity. During a median follow-up of nearly five years, 4,699 people had died. The worst long-term survival was observed in people of normal weight who displayed central obesity: a person with a BMI of 22 kg/m^2 who had a waist-to-hip ratio (WHR) of 0.98 had significantly higher mortality than a person with a similar BMI and a WHR of 0.89 (hazard ratio, 1.10); they also had significantly higher mortality than a person with a BMI of 30 kg/m^2 and WHR of 0.89 or 0.98 (hazard ratios, 1.61 and 1.27, respectively).[2]

A separate meta-analysis of several other studies, which looked at 16,000 patients, found that a high BMI correlated with a 35 percent

(continues)

(continued)

lower risk of death, but having a large waist in addition to a high BMI nearly doubled the risk of dying. To focus on waist size, the researchers controlled for age, hypertension, diabetes, and other risk factors for heart disease. Even heart patients with apple-shaped bodies and BMIs in the normal range were at increased risk of dying sooner, which drives home the fact that normal-weight heart patients may also need to lose some weight in their bellies. Bottom Line: Waist circumference seems to be a good indicator of cardiovascular risk.[3]

Along with a BMI calculator, I tell my patients to buy a tape measure and to measure their waist circumference. If your waist size is greater than your inseam you probably need to trim down a bit. The standard measurement for women is < 38 inches and men < 40 inches, though I think those numbers are a bit high a should be an inch or two lower.

ARE YOU AN APPLE OR A PEAR?

We've discussed that it's not just body fat percentage but also the distribution of that fat that puts us at risk for cardiovascular illness. It's been long held that people who are "apple-shaped"—usually men with more fat concentrated around the abdomen—are more at risk for heart disease and diabetes than their pear-shaped cousins, usually women who carry their weight in the hips, thighs and buttocks.

Recent study (see "Is a Pear Really the Fairer Fruit" below) notwithstanding about the role of gluteal fat as a precursor for metabolic syndrome, it's generally thought that having a pear shaped body is more protective against heart disease than an apple shape. Pear shaped women can expect to live up 9.5 years longer than their large waistline counterparts. The projections are even grimmer for

IS A PEAR REALLY THE FAIRER FRUIT?

Extending as far back as the Garden of Eden, the apple has gotten a bad rap. No one ever talks about a "bad pear" or a "rotten pear," though it is good to be the "apple of someone's eye." But having a pear shaped body may not be all it's cracked up to be and may, in fact, be more myth than reality.

Turns out that fat stored in the buttock area—known as gluteal adipose tissue—secretes abnormal levels of chemerin and omentin-1, proteins that can lead to inflammation and insulin resistance in people with early metabolic syndrome. The abnormal levels of these two proteins were also independent of age, body mass index and waist circumference. Gluteal fat, said the researchers, doesn't appear to protect against diabetes, heart disease, and metabolic syndrome and that the aforementioned abnormal protein levels may be an early way to spot those most at risk for developing metabolic syndrome.

Elevated levels of chemerin correlated with high blood pressure, elevated levels of C-reactive protein (a sign of inflammation) and triglycerides, insulin resistance, and low levels of HDL cholesterol, four of five indicators of metabolic syndrome. Low omentin-1 levels correlated with high levels of triglycerides and blood glucose levels and low levels of HDL cholesterol.

The good news, said the researchers, is that weight loss reduces chemerin levels along with other risk factors for metabolic syndrome.[4]

men, as a thirty-year-old with a beer belly can expect to die seventeen years before someone with a flat stomach.

But just why is it worse to be an apple than a pear? How is possible that body shape can predict our health destiny. Our body shape is determined by where we carry our fat. We find our shape by measuring your waist circumference and hip circumference, and then calculating your waist to hip ratio. .80 or above classifies you as an apple. Below .80 means you're a pear.

Apple-shaped folks store excess abdominal fat, which surrounds their organs and contributes to inflammation via C-reactive protein and an increase in blood sugar. Abdominal fat produces chemicals and hormones that make people more susceptible to heart disease, cancer, and diabetes. They're also more likely to have anxiety, depression, menstrual irregularities and fertility problems.

Pear-shaped people, on the other hand, collect weight around their hips, butt and thighs. Their fat is called subcutaneous fat. Subcutaneous/pear-zone fat is in the passive storage department. It stores fat as energy for release only in childbearing/breastfeeding, which explains why this sort of fat is found most often in women. It acts as fat magnet. Any fat we eat that we don't immediately need for energy is stored immediately *on the hips.* Pear-shaped women are more susceptible to problems like osteoporosis, varicose veins, and cellulite, and eating disorders stemming from poor self-esteem. Pear-shaped women also have less androgen (a male hormone effect that strengthens bones in apples), and at menopause, their pear-fat makes much weaker estrogen, which is not strong enough to keep calcium in the bones (apple fat produces estrogen during menopause, keeping the bones strong).

But hold the presses: Maybe body size doesn't matter as much as we thought. There have been challenges recently to the idea that being an apple puts you at greater risk than being a pear. A report published in the *Lancet* that pooled data from studies involving more than 220,000 people determined that conventional risk factors such as smoking, high blood pressure, and diabeters were accurate predictors of a heart attack or stroke but additional information about weight or body shape—ascertained by measuring waist circumference or waist-to-hip ratio—did not improve the ability to predict risk. As the study's co-author, Dr. Emanuele Di Angelantonio told the online journal *Heartwire,* "It has been thought that central adiposity (apple shape) is associated with a greater risk of cardiovascular disease than other types of obesity, but we have shown in our study that any one of three measures of obesity are equally associated with heart disease. So being an apple is no worse than being a pear. Both are bad."

Dr. Di Angelantonio wasn't saying that being an apple wasn't significant. Rather, he was making the point that that having an apple-shaped body doesn't put us at greater risk than other shapes, which is a shift from the zeitgeist. Ultimately, what is most important to understand? All forms of obesity are significant since each is linked to cardiovascular disease.

RESHAPING YOUR SHAPE WITH H-E-A-R-T

Whether you're an apple or a pear, if you're carrying around excess weight you're at risk for cardiovascular illness. Just a few pounds, or as little as two inches from your waistline can do wonders. You will reduce your chances by 50 percent or more of getting these diseases just by losing two inches.

If you're an apple:

1. Attack Adipose with Fiber-Rich Foods. They slow digestion of sugars, lower insulin and cholesterol levels and lower risk of heart disease and diabetes.

2. Energize with Aerobic Exercise. Thirty minutes daily is the easiest way to lose fat.

3. Reduce Blood Sugar and Tackle Triglycerides. If these tests are abnormal or even borderline, apples should be concerned and look into ways to remedy a possible problem.

If you're a pear:

1. Attack Adipose with Low-Fat Foods. Pear-zone fat cells are FAT magnets and will continue to store fat the more you consume, making your problem areas even worse, which can lead to poor body image or even eating disorders

2. Energize with Resistance Training. This type of exercise is great for pears to strengthen their bones

Since a higher BMI correlates with an increased risk of coronary artery disease, I recommend that you—whether or not you're at risk—calculate and keep track of yours. If you have CAD, I'd suggest you know both your BMI and waist size. Remember that central (abdominal) obesity is a more accurate predictor of disability and death than a high BMI.

I encourage you to "Act on Fat" because the data clearly show if you don't shape up it's likely you'll ship out.

CHAPTER 7

Blood Sugar:
Sweet Heart = Sour Health

In this chapter you'll learn the forth step in following your heart by "R—reducing your blood sugar."

Doctors know that high blood sugar levels are bad for the heart. In fact, the connection between diabetes and heart disease starts with high blood glucose, as people with diabetes are two to four times more likely to develop cardiovascular illness. In this chapter, I explain how high blood sugar puts people at risk for developing cardiovascular disease, and look at the reasons why, in an age where millions of diabetics worldwide use synthetic insulin to regulate their blood sugar levels, diabetes is still skyrocketing. Drawing on the experience of hundreds of my patients, I've created an aggressive, proactive program to lower blood sugar levels and cut the risk of cardiovascular disease. "Dreadful outcomes are optional," I tell patients. Indeed, as this chapter demonstrates, diabetes is unique among chronic diseases in that it's a condition where we can almost always change course without invasive medical intervention and put ourselves on the path to optimal heart health.

A LIFE-SAVING BEE STING: MARY'S STORY

Mary was nothing if not a hard worker. Indeed, she didn't think twice about coming to her office early and staying long after everyone else had left for the day. But Mary truly loved her job as an assistant director of marketing at a major women's clothing label and really didn't mind the long hours. At age fifty, with both of her children grown and off to college, and her husband traveling frequently on business, she had discovered a renewed passion for her work. She loved everything about her job, particularly the annual office picnic, which took place every year at a beautiful, seaside estate not far from her home.

It was a hot July afternoon when Mary decided to exchange her heels for a pair of flip-flops and take a walk along the beach with two colleagues. On this day, Mary didn't notice a bee circling around a small honeysuckle near the bench where she was changing shoes. Predictably, she got too close and the bee proceeded to sting Mary on her left foot. Immediately, Mary's foot started to swell. Strangely enough, she felt nothing. Then Mary felt the bee still on her foot, repeatedly and violently injecting its stinger into her heel. Still, Mary barely noticed it. It didn't hurt, even a little. In fact, she was numb, feeling nothing at all. Mary found the whole incident odd since she'd been stung by bees and wasps many times before and it *always* hurt.

Mary didn't think much about the incident and went about enjoying the party, even going for a walk, her swollen foot notwithstanding. That night Mary called her husband, who'd been traveling, to tell him what happened. He was concerned. "Bee stings usually hurt like hell," he told her. "Maybe you should see a doctor."

Two days later, Mary is sitting on the exam table, her doctor carefully inspecting her left foot. The swelling has subsided, but Mary told her doctor that she still felt nothing. "The bee must've have stung me five, maybe six times and I have to be honest, I didn't feel a thing. It didn't even hurt. Maybe, I'm immune," she joked.

But to Mary's doctor this was no laughing matter. He started asking her questions. "Have you felt any tingling in your foot, or any of your extremities for that matter?" he asked. In fact, Mary had noticed "pins and needles" in her feet and hands, but simply attributed it to long hours behind a desk without a break. "Maybe I need to get up a walk around during the day more," she offered.

The doctor pressed on. "Do you have burning or stabbing pains in your feet? Do your feet get very hot or cold for no reason?" "That happened for a while," answered Mary, adding that she had brushed the whole thing aside, thinking it was something that would just go away on its own. One thing that Mary had noticed was that her feet felt "dead." "They seem weak and sometimes I have trouble standing or walking," she continued. Of great concern to the doctor was a single open sore, accompanied by an abundant amount of dry, cracked skin, on the bottom of Mary's right foot. "How long have you had that sore?" asked the doctor. "I didn't even know I had a cut on the bottom of my foot," replied Mary.

The doctor had heard enough. Based on her symptoms, recent medical history, as well as his own physical exam, he suspected that Mary had peripheral neuropathy, a form of nerve damage that frequently occurs in people with diabetes. Depending on the affected nerves, symptoms of diabetic neuropathy can range from pain and numbness in the extremities to problems with the digestive system, urinary tract, blood vessels, and even the heart. For some people, these symptoms are mild; for others, they can be disabling and even fatal.

The doctor ordered a full battery of tests, including nerve conduction studies to measure how quickly the nerves in Mary's legs were conducting electrical signals. Also, the tests would rule out other illness with similar symptoms such as Parkinson's, multiple sclerosis and other autoimmune diseases, all of which can compromise the integrity of the nerves. Although peripheral neuropathy can have many causes, diabetes is the number one risk factor. So along with the neurological testing, Mary's doctor ordered blood work, including two separate glycated hemoglobin (A1C) tests, which would indicate Mary's average blood sugar level for the preceding two to three months, and a random blood sugar test. The GH test measures the percentage of blood sugar attached to hemoglobin, the oxygen-carrying protein in red blood cells. The higher your blood sugar levels, the more hemoglobin you'll have with sugar attached. Mary's A1C level of 7.0 percent on two separate tests confirmed that she had type 2 diabetes, normal for someone entering midlife. As a rule, any blood sugar levels out of the normal range could signify diabetes.

Peripheral neuropathy is a long-term, serious complication of diabetes. And the nerve impairment occurs after prolonged exposure to the damaging effects of high blood glucose levels. Though diabetic neuropathy most often attacks the nerves in the legs and feet, high blood sugar can injure nerve fibers throughout the body. Simply, the longer a person has diabetes, the higher the risk of developing neuropathy. Mary didn't even know she was so sick.

Mary was lucky. The doctor informed her that could slow the progress of her illness with tight blood sugar control and a healthy lifestyle.

AN EPIDEMIC WITH NO SIGN OF SLOWING DOWN

Diabetes is ubiquitous. That shouldn't come as a shock. I know few people whose lives haven't been touched in some way by diabetes. The numbers are alarming. Diabetes is the third leading disease-related cause of death in the United States. According to the most recent statistics compiled by the National Institutes of Health (NIH), which cover through 1996, there were 10.3 million diagnosed diabetics in America, and approximately 5.5 million who have diabetes but haven't yet been diagnosed. This number has no doubt increased. Nearly 800,000 new diabetics will be diagnosed this year alone, according to NIH statistics. That's three new cases every two minutes.[1]

More alarming, perhaps, is that type 2 diabetes—once called adult-onset diabetes—is prevalent among children. In 2002, a Yale University study that looked at obese children between the ages four and eighteen found that nearly a quarter had a condition that's often a precursor to diabetes. Since then, obesity rates among children have skyrocketed, and so has the incidence of type 2 diabetes. Even more frightening, a recent study by researchers at Massachusetts General Hospital found diabetes progresses faster in children than in adults and is harder to treat.

Tens of thousands of Americans lose their eyesight annually because of diabetes; the leading cause of new blindness for people ages twenty-five to seventy-four. Ninety-five percent of diabetics have type 2 diabetes.

DIABETES: THE BASICS

The ancient Greeks described diabetes as a disease that causes the body to melt into sugar water. This is an accurate description. Diabetes, often referred to by doctors as diabetes mellitus, is a group of metabolic diseases in which the person has high blood glucose (blood sugar) resulting from inadequate insulin production, failure of the body's cells to respond properly to insulin, or both. Diabetes is insidious; there is probably not a tissue in the body that escapes the effects of chronically elevated blood sugar. Side effects of high blood sugar include osteoporosis, frequent urination, increased thirst, tight, wrinkled skin (which takes place by process known as crosslinking) or dry, itchy skin, inflammation and arthritis, and impaired short-term memory.

INSULIN: THE BASICS

No discussion of diabetes is possible without first mentioning the pancreas, a hand-sized gland located toward the back of the abdominal cavity. The pancreas is a true multi-tasker but it's primarily responsible for manufacturing, storing, and releasing insulin, a hormone. Insulin regulates the amount of glucose in our bloodstream, which it does through a very precise system that stimulates something I'll refer to as "glucose transporters" to move to the surface of cells, which facilitates the entry of glucose into the cells. This is critical since glucose is our cells primary food source. Insulin then stimulates the hypothalamus, and the part of the brain responsible for feeding behavior. Insulin also signals fat cells to convert glucose and fatty acids from the blood into fat, which the fat cells then store until needed. Insulin is an anabolic hormone, meaning it's responsible for the growth of many tissues and organs. Insulin helps to regulate, or counter-regulate, the balance of certain other hormones in the body. One of the ways insulin maintains the narrow range of normal levels of glucose in the blood is by regulation of the liver and muscles, directing them to manufacture and store glycogen, a starchy substance the body calls upon when blood sugar falls too low. When the body exhausts its supply of glucose and glycogen, the liver, and to a lesser extent the kidneys and small intestines, kick into high gear, transforming some of the body's protein stores—muscle mass and vital organs—into glucose. Excess insulin can lead to increased body fat and the rapid growth of cells that line blood our vessels. Insulin stimulates the uptake of glucose (sugar) from the blood to the cells in the body. When the body's cells are resistant to the action of the insulin, as in the case of obesity and the metabolic syndrome, the body creates more insulin resulting in hyperinsulinemia, which, along with insulin resistance, causes a myriad of problems including:

- High triglycerides (increased risk of heart and stroke)
- High plasminogen activator inhibitor activity (PAI-Fx), causing increased risk of clotting
- low HDL cholesterol (increased risk of heart attack and stroke)

- high uric acid (gout)
- polycystic ovary syndrome (endocrine disorder with oligo-amenorrhea, infertility, hirsutism, obesity, high Leptin levels
- type 2 diabetes
- obesity

High insulin can also stimulate the kidney to produce angiotension, a substance that increases blood pressure.

Insulin resistance syndrome promotes:

- heart attack
- stroke
- type 2 diabetes
- morbid obesity
- hypertension
- endocrine disorders in women
- clotting problems
- Polycystic ovarian syndrome

Hyperinsulinemia (too much insulin) is a significant independent risk factor for coronary heart disease and directly impacts how the lining of the blood vessels responds to changes in blood pressure. These effects are separate from the other dangerous effects on fat composition and blood pressure. Treating insulin resistance syndrome can significantly reduce the health risks as summarized above.

THE THREE-HEADED MONSTER

There are three types of diabetes: type 1, type 2, and gestational diabetes. Though the locus of this book's efforts is type 2 diabetes, a little background might be helpful since all three yield similar side effects. Almost 200,000 people die annually from both type 1 and type 2 diabetes. I suspect that number is much higher since diabetics develop other illness that may be listed as the cause of death but never would have occurred if they hadn't been initiated by diabetes.

TYPE 1 DIABETES

Just a decade ago, before the clinical availability of insulin, a diagnosis of type 1-diabetes—which involves a severely diminished or complete inability to produce insulin—was a death sentence. Most people died within a few months of diagnosis. Why? Without insulin, glucose accumulates in the blood at extremely toxic levels. And since the cells cannot utilize glucose many simply starve. Absent or lowered fasting (basal) levels of insulin also lead the liver, kidneys, and intestines to perform gluconeogenesis, turning the body's protein store—the muscles and vital organs—into even more glucose that the body cannot utilize. Meanwhile, the kidneys, whose job it are to filter our blood, try to rid the body of these inappropriately high levels of sugar. Frequent urination causes insatiable thirst and dehydration. Eventually, the starving body turns more and more protein to sugar.

When tissues cannot utilize glucose, they will metabolize fat for energy, generating by-products called ketones, which are toxic at high levels and cause further water loss as the kidneys try to eliminate them.

Today, type 1 diabetes is still a very serious disease, and fatal if not properly treated with insulin. It may kill quickly—imagine a rapid drop in blood sugar (hypoglycemia) that impairs your judgment or causes a loss of consciousness while operating a motor vehicle—or it may kill inexorably by heart or kidney disease, which are commonly associated with long-term blood sugar elevation. The exact cause of type 1 diabetes is still unknown. Research seems to point in the direction of an autoimmune disorder. In this instance, the body's immune system attacks pancreatic beta cells, which produce insulin. It may be hard to prevent type 1 diabetes, but the earlier it's diagnosed, and blood sugars are brought under control, the better off you'll be.

TYPE 2 DIABETES: THE SELF-INFLICTED WOUND

Medically speaking, type 2 diabetes is a less serious illness. But type 2 diabetes is an insidious disease, weaving its web via chronically but less alarmingly elevated blood sugars levels. Because type 2 diabetes affects an estimated 25.8 million people (8.3 percent of the U.S. population and I believe an underreported figure), it causes more problems long term that its type 1 counterpart. The American Diabetes Association estimates that 90–95 percent of diabetics are type 2. Hypertension, heart disease, kidney failure, blindness, and erectile dysfunction result directly or indirectly from type 2 diabetes. Type 2 often progresses unabated because it's milder and thus left untreated or treated badly.

Unlike type 1 diabetics, type 2 sufferers make insulin. Left untreated, however, type 2 diabetes strain pancreatic beta cells, whose job it is to store and release insulin, and affects insulin's ability to reduce blood glucose concentrations. Beta cells can respond quickly to blood glucose spikes by secreting stored insulin while simultaneously producing more, making supplemental insulin necessary.

Did you know that an early sign of mild chronic blood sugar elevation in women is recurrent vaginal yeast infections?

Type 2 diabetes is the far more prevalent of the two. Numbers vary but as many as a quarter of Americans between the ages of sixty-five and seventy-four have type 2 diabetes. Even kids are feeling the effects. A Yale University study found that 25 percent of obese teenagers now have type 2 diabetes.

THE NEW DIABETES

There's a new kid on the block. Latent autoimmune diabetes, or LADA, is a mild form of diabetes (sometimes referred to as "pre-diabetes") that appears after age thirty-five. With LADA, an antibody is produced to a pancreatic beta cell protein called GADA, just as in the case of type 1 diabetes. LADA sufferers can develop full-blown diabetes and require insulin.[2]

Roughly 80 percent of type 2 diabetics are overweight or obese, with most of that weight concentrated around the abdomen. The remaining 20 percent who don't have visceral obesity may actually have a mild form of type 1 diabetes, resulting in only a partial loss of insulin producing pancreatic beta cells. If this is true, then a majority of type 2 diabetics may be overweight.

Unlike type 1 diabetes, there's little doubt as to the origins of type 2 diabetes. Indeed, there's a reason type 2 diabetes is also known as "insulin-resistant diabetes." Obesity and insulin resistance—the inability to fully utilize the glucose-transporting effects of insulin—go hand-in-hand. A study in the *Journal of Clinical Investigation* concluded "…insulin resistance, in addition to being caused by obesity, can contribute to the development of obesity."[3]

Fat in muscles cells, known as intramyocyte fat, is a contributing factor in the development of insulin resistance.

Insulin resistance appears to be caused at least in part by inheritance. A rare but severe condition known as Inherited Insulin Resistance Syndrome stems from a mutation in the insulin receptor gene. Whatever its source, insulin resistance increases the body's need for insulin, causing the pancreas to work harder to produce elevated insulin levels (the aforementioned hyperinsulinemia), which we know triggers hypertension and damages the circulatory system. Hyperinsulinemia also creates "tolerance" to insulin's message, causing even greater insulin resistance.

THE OTHER CULPRIT IN INSULIN RESISTANCE

Triglycerides circulate in our bloodstream at all times. High triglyceride levels come more from carbohydrate consumption and existing body fat then they do from a high intake of dietary fat. How do we know this? Carbohydrates are converted to glucose, our body's preferred energy source. Whatever glucose isn't used immediately gets processed by the liver and converted into glycogen, which is stored in muscle tissue. Insufficient muscle mass coupled with excess glycogen triggers the liver to process glucose again, only this time into triglycerides, explaining why the majority of fat in our bodies are triglycerides. Our bodies use them for energy if glucose isn't available.

Whenever I see a patient with high blood sugar, I know that he or she will most likely have elevated triglycerides. The reason is simple: Insulin removes triglycerides from our bloodstream, which is why high triglycerides can be an early indication of insulin resistance or even diabetes.

BLOOD SUGAR

High blood sugar is a hallmark of diabetes, and the cause of every long-term complication of the disease. Thus, a discussion of where blood sugar comes from and how it is used seems helpful.

Carbohydrates and proteins are our dietary source of sugar. And we love sugar. Why not? It tastes great, in part because it fosters the creation of neurotransmitters that relieve anxiety and can even create a sense of well-being or euphoria. No wonder some people have carb cravings that take on an addictive quality. Low blood sugar levels cause the liver, kidneys, and intestines to convert proteins into

---

COULD HIGH BLOOD SUGAR REALLY BE ALL IN YOUR HEAD?

We all know that high blood sugar is bad for our heart. But now a new study suggests that people with high blood sugar, even if they don't have diabetes, are at added risk for developing Alzheimer's disease.

The study, which tracked blood sugar over time in people with and without diabetes, found that every incremental increase in blood sugar was associated with a higher risk of dementia. The results of the study suggest that controlling blood sugar levels is important for staving off cognitive decline. Just as with heart disease, the risk of dementia rises as blood sugar does. And just as exercising and controlling blood pressure, blood sugar, and cholesterol are a viable ways to delay or prevent heart disease, they appear to do the same for dementia.[4]

---

glucose, but very slowly and inefficiently. The body cannot convert glucose back into protein, nor can it convert fat into sugar. Fat cells, however, with the help of insulin, do transform glucose into fat.

How important is it to control blood sugar? The Diabetes Control and Complication Trial (DCCT), conducted by the NIH's National Institute of Diabetes and Digestive and Kidney Diseases (NIDDK), was first set up to gauge the effects of improved control of blood sugar levels in type 1 diabetics. Patients whose blood sugars were nearly "normalized" had dramatic reductions of long-term complications. For example, researchers discovered that controlling blood sugar led to a 75 percent reduction in the progression of early diabetic retinopathy. They found similarly dramatic results with other diabetes complications including kidney disease, a reduction of risk for nerve damage, and a 35 percent reduction of risk for cardiovascular disease.

The patients followed in the DCCT averaged twenty-seven years of age at the beginning of the trial, so reductions could easily have been greater in areas such as cardiovascular disease if they had been older or followed for a longer period of time. The implication is that full normalization of blood sugar could totally prevent these complications. In any case, the results of the DCCT are good reason to begin aggressively to monitor and normalize blood sugar levels.

ON THE HORIZON

The best bet for controlling diabetes is normalizing your blood sugars. Sounds simple enough. But most things in life are easier said than done.

There is research underway that would allow scientists to replicate insulin-producing pancreatic beta cells in the laboratory. In theory, this would cure diabetes, allowing anyone to remain free of the disease for life. Another potential approach might involve the insertion of the genes for insulin production into liver or kidney cells. This tactic has successfully cured diabetes in rats but hasn't been tested in humans.

But these approaches, while potentially helpful, fail to address an important component of high blood sugar.

USING H-E-A-R-T TO REIGN IN HIGH BLOOD SUGAR

Because there are rarely any symptoms from diabetes until it has become seriously advanced, monitoring blood sugar and sugar in the urine are the only ways of detecting this serious, even life threatening disease. It is a known fact that being overweight increases our risk of diabetes and it is also known that the majority of diabetes can be prevented by changes in lifestyle. I tell my patients who are overweight and at risk for diabetes that exercise is the most important part of achieving and maintaining optimal cardiovascular health. I often quote a study by the Diabetes Prevention Program showing how more than 3,000 people at high risk for diabetes delayed and even prevented the disease by losing a small amount of weight (5 to 7 percent of total body weight) through thirty minutes of physical activity five days a week and healthier eating.

STRESS AND BLOOD SUGAR

From weight gain to cardiovascular illness, stress seems to be front and center of any number of chronic diseases. Now it seems that people under high stress have something else to worry about: high blood sugar levels.

Think about what happens to your body during times of stress. Your breath becomes shallow, your pulse quickens, and your stomach hurts. Stress also triggers the release of glucose—sugar—from the liver, a way of preparing the body to take action—the infamous "fight or flight response."

But this response to stress was meant to be short term. How often do you find yourself in fight or flight situations? When was the last time you had to run from a rabid dog? A lousy job, a troubled marriage, health concerns, financial struggles—chronic stress is the stress that vexes us most. Problem is that our body doesn't distinguish between the two. The "fight or flight" response occurs with both. Any ongoing anxiety can trigger a stress response. Chronic stress is not healthy, but it's especially awful for anyone with high blood sugar because additional glucose is being continually released into your bloodstream. This glucose is *in addition to* what we take in from food.

The good news: Simple relaxation exercises and other stress management techniques, such as my BREATHE TECHNIQUE™ can help you gain more control over blood sugar levels. A study at Duke University found that people with high blood sugar levels who took five diabetes-education classes with stress-management training improved their blood sugar levels enough to lower their risk of the most serious complications, including heart disease, kidney failure, nerve damage, and vision problems.[5]

I tell all my patients that regular exercise is key to following your H-E-A-R-T because exercise helps heal your blood pressure, energize your heart, acts against fat, reduces blood sugar, and helps tackle triglycerides all at the same time.

CHAPTER 8

Cholesterol: The Skinny on Fat

In this chapter you'll learn the fifth step to follow your heart by "T—Tackling triglycerides."

Did you know that President Dwight D. Eisenhower was obsessed with lowering his cholesterol? So much so that he took extreme measures to remove fat from his diet. It didn't do much good, apparently, as his blood cholesterol kept climbing, and he eventually died of heart disease. These days, we're just as obsessed. In medical circles, cholesterol is the big "C" word. Everywhere you turn, there's another news story or medical alert about the importance of paying attention to our cholesterol and triglyceride levels. But what does this really mean? After all, cholesterol and triglycerides are essential for our well-being. Indeed, they are necessary for life itself. In this chapter, I'm going to demystify fat; answering the questions I'm asked every day in my practice, in the media, and following lectures. I'll tell you everything you need to know about these critical fats, breakdown the cholesterol/heart disease connection, particularly as it relates to the development of atherosclerosis, the disease most responsible for life threatening cardiovascular events; and tell you what you can do to tackle and optimize your cholesterol and triglyceride levels, not through medications or invasive surgical intervention, but thorough cutting-edge diet, exercise, and stress reduction tools critical for optimal heart health.

HYPERCHOLESTEROLEMIA: ANNA'S STORY

Nothing could slow Anna down. As a busy kindergarten teacher and mother of two young children, she was used to being on the go. Indeed, five days a week she was up in the morning at 5:30 and seldom did she turn in before 11 P.M.

One day while getting dressed for work, Anna noticed a small but conspicuous bump on her left Achilles' tendon just above her heel. Anna, who was a college track standout and still found time for a daily 5-K trek, spent minutes marveling at the tendon's symmetry, width and thickness, following its course to her calf muscle, at which point she discovered the same lump above her right heel. The following night Anna was climbing the three flights of stairs to her apartment, just as she'd done hundreds of times before. Suddenly, and without warning, crushing, oppressive chest pain gripped Anna and she collapsed. Anna's landlord, who was outside watering some plants, witnessed the event. Fortunately, he had some medical training, called 911, and rushed over. Immediately, he started shaking and shouting at Anna, and rubbed her sternum with his knuckles, a technique that could help determine the cause of her collapse. Anne was unresponsive, which is often the case with cardiac arrest, so the landlord immediately began chest compression and mouth-to-mouth CPR. Paramedics arrived within minutes and not a second to soon since Anna still didn't have a pulse. She received two shocks from a defibrillator, which delivers a therapeutic dose of electrical energy to the heart. Defibrillation is the definitive treatment for life-threatening conditions such as cardiac arrhythmias, ventricular fibrillation, and pulseless ventricular tachycardia.

Paramedics restored Anna's pulse and she was rushed to the emergency room, where I performed an emergency angioplasty and stenting on her blocked coronary artery. I diagnosed Anna with *familial combined hyperlipidemia*, meaning as its name implies, an inherited disorder of high cholesterol and high blood triglycerides. Familial combined hyperlipidemia is the most common genetic disorder of increased blood fat(s) that leads to early heart attacks. Thus far, we haven't a clue as to the specific genes responsible.

While Anna recovered in the ICU, I learned that her father, as well as all her paternal uncles had heart attacks in their thirties and accompanying thick Achilles tendons, a condition known medically as *tendinous xanthomas*, and a common clinical finding in those with familial hyperlipidemia.

As a former college track champ and self-described "healthy person," Anna wondered how she could suffer cardiac arrest. Moreover, she seemed baffled that a thick Achilles tendon, the sort seen in well-conditioned athletes and dancers and coveted by weightlifters and body sculpting aficionados, almost ended her life. What's the thick tendon-high cholesterol connection all about?

A xanthoma is a cholesterol-filled yellow-colored nodule or bump that's found just under skin or along tendons. Xanthomas look harmless but their presence is a strong indicator of high blood (LDL) cholesterol, which significantly increases the risk of cardiovascular disease, including the advanced atherosclerosis that nearly killed Anna.

Xanthomas are found around the inner or outer areas of the eyelids, where they often occur in clusters; around joints (especially on the elbows or knees), in the creases of the palms and fingers, on the feet and on the buttocks, and within tendons that travel along the backs of the hands and arms, the tops of the feet or within the Achilles tendon on the heel, as was the case with Anna. People who eat a high-fat, low-fiber diet, are overweight, and do not get sufficient exercise are susceptible to xanthomas, but none of these risk factors applied to Anna. Her only risk factor was IFH, which begins in early childhood and where it probably started for Anna. Xanthomas are unsightly; particularly those that occur around the eye, and many people have them removed by a dermatologic or plastic surgeon. But far more important than its removal, is prompt attention to the high blood cholesterol that caused it in the first place.

What can we learn from Anna's brush with death? Bottom Line: High cholesterol kills. Having said that, I'll admit that's also a simplistic way of looking at things given cholesterol's essential role in human well-being. That's why getting a handle on the problem demands that you know the skinny on this important fat.

CHOLESTEROL: TESTING YOUR KNOWLEDGE OF THE SKINNY ON FAT

Here's a question: What do you know about cholesterol and triglycerides? Reciting what they read in magazines or repeating an admonition from their doctors during an annual physical, most people would say that elevated cholesterol and triglycerides are a serious health problem. They would be right, of course. Indeed, high cholesterol and triglycerides affect an estimated fifty million Americans. Elevated cholesterol and triglycerides are a major risk factor for cardiovascular disease. Everywhere you turn, there's another news story or medical alert about the importance of paying attention to cholesterol and triglyceride levels. But what does this really mean? After all, in and of themselves, these fats aren't bad. While high cholesterol and triglyceride levels can be harmful, just the right amount is critical for normal body functioning. You couldn't live without them. Yet, these fats have gotten a bad rap and remain poorly understood, leaving many confused as to their role in human wellbeing.

WHAT IS CHOLESTEROL?

Cholesterol is a fat. This point should be obvious from the chapter title alone. But as Juliet recited in that famous play, "What's in a name?" sometimes the names of things don't matter, only what things are. And what is cholesterol? To begin, cholesterol is a naturally occurring sterol, or steroid alcohol found in both plants and animals and from which the aptly titled "steroid" hormones are made. Cholesterol is waxy—think melted candle—and a whitish /yellowish colored substance that flows through the body via the blood. And here's where things get tricky. Because cholesterol is oil-based and blood is water-based, cholesterol can't simply be dumped into your bloodstream. To get a visual picture of this concept, try dropping cooking oil into a glass of water. Notice how the oil floats on the surface instead of mixing? Now imagine that oil-based cholesterol in your bloodstream. It would congeal into unusable globs. Our bodies get around this transportation problem by packaging cholesterol and other fats into minuscule protein-covered particles called lipoproteins (lipid + protein), which mix easily with blood, and are critical for any discussion about heart disease.

The fat in these particles is made up of cholesterol, triglycerides, and phospholipids. Triglycerides compose about 90 percent of the fat in the food we eat. We need triglycerides for energy, but too much of these good things are bad for our hearts.

HDL AND LDL: KNOWING THE DIFFERENCE

Low-density lipoproteins (LDL) and high-density lipoproteins (HDL) sound similar but they're as different as a turnip and a tow truck. The differences stem from their densities; particles with more fat and less protein (LDL) have a lower density than their high-protein, low-fat counterparts (HDL). LDL and HDL are best to get a basic understanding of how cholesterol affects your body and how the food you eat affects your cholesterol levels.

LOW DENSITY LIPOPORTEIN (LDL)

In the world of cholesterol, LDL is a double-edged sword. LDL cholesterol is manufactured in the liver, and up to 70 percent of the

SATURATED VS UNSATURATED FAT: A PRIMER[1]

Everyone talks about saturated and unsaturated fat. But what does all that really mean? To simplify matters, I've created this easy to follow chart for quick reference.

	Saturated Fats	Unsaturated Fats
Type of bonds:	Consist of single hydrogen bond (meaning they're evenly filled out with hydrogen)	Consist of at least 1 DOUBLE bond resulting in a polyunsaturated fatty acid
Recommended consumption:	Less than 10percent of total calories per day	Up to 30percent of total calories per day
Health Effects:	Excessive consumption is not good because of their association with atherosclerosis and heart diseases.	Unsaturated fats are considered good to eat if you are watching your cholesterol.
Cholesterol:	Saturated fats increase LDL (bad cholesterol) and decrease the HDL (good cholesterol)	Unsaturated fats increase high-density lipoprotein (HDL or good cholesterol) and decrease LDL (bad cholesterol)
Commonly found in:	Butter, coconut oil, whole milk, meat, peanut butter, margarine, cheese, vegetable oil or fish oil	Avocado, soybean oil, canola oil and olive oil
Shelf Life:	These are long lasting and do not get spoiled quickly	These get spoiled quickly
Melting Point:	High	Low
Physical state at room temperature:	Solid	Liquid
Rancidity:	Low	High
Examples:	Bacon, butter	Olive Oil

body's cholesterol is carried by LDL particles to where it's needed most. LDL is a critical building block of cell walls, hormones, and digestive juices. Yet, too much LDL, especially small particle LDL, greatly increases the risk for CAD since excess amounts of it deposit in our arteries, causing blockages that could lead to heart attacks. The amount of LDL in your bloodstream is related to the amount of saturated fat and cholesterol you eat, which is why people with elevated LDL cholesterol are encouraged to follow a reduced-fat diet. If you follow my recommendations outlined at the end of this chapter then you'll have some idea of numbers needed to optimal heart health.

HIGH DENSITY LIPOPROTEIN (HDL)

HDL is basically the opposite of LDL. Instead of having a lot of fat, HDL has gobs of protein. Instead of transporting cholesterol around the body, HDL is the body's version of Pac Man, gobbling up as much excess cholesterol as it can. It picks up extra cholesterol from the cells and tissues and also transports it back to the liver, which takes the cholesterol out of the particle and either uses it to make bile or recycles it. This action partially explains why high levels of HDL are thought to be beneficial and associated with low risk for heart disease. HDL also contains antioxidant molecules that may prevent LDL from being changed into a lipoprotein that is even more likely to cause heart disease. Lifestyle changes affect HDL levels—exercise can increase them, while obesity and smoking lower them. As for diet, in general, the high-fat diets that raise LDL also raise HDL, while low-fat diets lower both. However, by carefully choosing the right foods, you can eat a diet that lowers LDL without lowering HDL, as I'll discuss in Chapter 9.

WHY YOU NEED CHOLESTEROL

Most doctors discuss cholesterol's role in our bodies. Just as often, I do the opposite, telling patients what could happen without cholesterol. A rare but serious genetic illness, *Smith-Lemli-Opitz Syndrome or SLOS*, occurs in people who can't make enough cholesterol on their own. People with full-blown SLOS inherit a defective gene for cholesterol synthesis from both of their biological parents. While just a small percentage of the population has this trait, it's so serious that it often leads to spontaneous abortion. And in this instances where a baby is born with SLOS, there's increased risk of a wide range of defects such as autism, compromised immune function, physical defects, digestive disorders, visual problems and mental retardation. Clearly, cholesterol is critical for human functioning.

What accounts for this little lipid molecule's profound effect? Trillions of cells compose our bodies. No exaggeration. And these trillions of cells need to interact with each other. Cholesterol is one of the molecules that allow these interactions to take place! Cholesterol, as an example, synthesizes bile acids in the liver, which are needed for the absorption of fat from the intestine, which explains why insufficient amounts of cholesterol adversely impact digestion.

Cholesterol also plays an essential role in our brains, not coincidentally the body's most cholesterol-rich organ. Cholesterol plays a leading role in synapse formation, or the connection between your neurons, and the vehicle that allows for data processing and memory function. Cholesterol, in fact, is so vital for proper brain function that a study out of Iowa State University found that statins, which inhibit the liver from making cholesterol, might also keep the brain from making cholesterol.

STATINS: MORE HARM THAN HELP?

Mona was distressed. As an attorney with a blue chip firm specializing in mergers & acquisitions, she was venerated around the office for her photographic memory. But now at age forty-nine, she was sitting in my exam room complaining that she couldn't recall where she'd left her purse, much less remember all the details involved in the buying, selling, dividing, and combining of different companies. "Maybe I should I see a neurologist, Dr. Kennedy. I think I may have dementia." Though you'd think Mona would be better off with a neurologist, she wasn't the first person I'd seen in my office recently complaining of memory problems. The thing Mona and my other patients had in common was statins. All had developed memory problems after taking statins (and in many cases the symptoms subsided and even improved after they stopped taking the medication).

Since they were first introduced in 1987, statins have transformed cardiac medicine. But like all drugs, statins come with considerable risks. Cognitive impairment is a widely reported side effect of statins but there are others, including muscle pain and damage, liver damage, digestive problems, rashes, elevated blood sugar and even type 2 diabetes. But the neurological deficits, particularly the memory loss and/or confusion, are especially distressing to patients. As a colleague of mine is fond of saying, "If you don't have your mental health, you don't have anything."

There is some irony in the fact that the one thing that makes statins helpful—their ability to inhibit the liver from synthesizing cholesterol so less of the substance is carried to the cells, thus lowering LDL cholesterol—is the thing that may harm brain function. But there may be some merit to it since, in accordance with FDA requirements, drug manufacturers must report any adverse events that they know about, and most statin bottles list memory loss and confusion as possible side effects. Studies have tied statins to aggressive, even violent behavior.[2] But here's the

(continues)

(continued)

$64,000 question: Was it the statin, diabetes, or an underlying cerebro-vascular disease that increased the risk for these patients?

What I know is that statins have been shown to prevent heart attacks from occurring in people at risk and second-time heart attacks in those already with disease, which is why I feel so strongly about statins. To ease the burden on patients and increase the efficacy of a drug, I typically switch from one statin to another. If side effects persist following a formal neurological exam, then I'll discontinue the drug for a month. If the side effects still don't improve, I make sure a patient and his loved ones have enough information to make an informed decision about whether or not to continue this form of treatment. Always, I'm careful to spell out the enormous benefit of statins.

As someone who prescribes statins almost daily, I think the jury is still out as to their effect on memory. And to my knowledge, all known clinical trials on statin use have never turned up memory problems, even in elderly patients (researchers once held hopes that the drugs might actually prevent cognitive decline and one study in fact suggested a 43 percent decreased risk).[3] Most patients taking statins have a greater risk of developing cognitive decline from heart disease, which can impair blood flow to the brain, than from drugs. All of this explains why the whole subject of statins is so confusing and quite frankly so easy to forget. As a cardiologist, what I can't forget is that well designed studies have shown statins to decrease first- and second-time heart attacks, lower rates of surgery, and decrease risk of death from CAD.

Yet, I've seen enough anecdotal evidence to believe that the effect isn't incidental. If you're taking statins and experiencing memory problems, speak with your doctor. Never go off your statin without first seeking medical advice. Short-term memory, like the sort Mona experienced, seems to be most affected by statins. Just don't start panicking if you misplace your keys.

CHOLESTEROL AND THE RISK OF HEART DISEASE: ANOTHER THEORY

Is conventional medicine seriously confused when it comes to cholesterol? There are some who believe that cardiovascular disease isn't the result of too much cholesterol but the human body's way of compensating for cholesterol sulfate deficiency. The theory goes that the body corrects for this imbalance by transforming LDL cholesterol into plaque, enabling blood platelets to produce the cholesterol sulfate the heart needs for optimal function. Under this scenario, high LDL—a known risk factor—is the body's signal that it needs to produce cholesterol sulfate. Thus, removing the LDL via statin drugs or other artificial mechanism, may also remove your body's "backup" mechanism to keep your heart as healthy as possible.

This represents a common "feedback" system when there is excess of something the body attempts to compensate by decreasing production to normalize and vice versa. I think the concept is interesting, though it's hard to argue against cholesterol being a very bad actor as it is invariably part of atherosclerotic plaque.

Yes, we need cholesterol.

Cholesterol is needed for many important synthetic functions and helps preserve and protect our brain and nervous system for example. Though cholesterol is likely a bad actor in the atherosclerotic process and invariably part of the heart-attack-causing plaque. There is a delicate balance between just how much or too little cholesterol is required to halt atherosclerosis yet maintain bodily functions. In cases of severely elevated cholesterol where levels sometimes exceed 500 or 1,000, the severity of coronary artery disease is often directly related. On the other hand, cholesterol levels that are too low can cause problems with the brain, nervous system and digestive system.

DOES THE BODY MAKE CHOLESTEROL?

Mother Nature is one smart cookie. She doesn't leave anything to chance. Our bodies have evolved to manufacture their own cholesterol, and don't have to rely on diet alone. Even if you ate a cholesterol-free diet, which is not such an easy thing to do, your body would make the 1,000 mg it needs to function properly. Your body regulates the amount of cholesterol in the blood, producing more when your diet doesn't provide adequate amounts. Cholesterol synthesis is a tightly controlled process.

Mason D. Freeman, M.D., a professor at Harvard Medical School, explained our body's cholesterol manufacturing process best in his important book, *The Harvard Medical School Guide to Lowering Your Cholesterol.* Dr. Freeman said the system works "much as your thermostat and furnace work to regulate the temperature in your home. The thermostat in this case is a protein that can sense the cholesterol content of a cell. When it senses a low level of cellular cholesterol, the protein signals the genes of the cell (the furnace in this analogy) to produce the proteins that make cholesterol. The cell makes more cholesterol, and it also makes more proteins on the cell surface that can capture the circulating LDL particles, thereby retrieving cholesterol by bringing it in from the blood." It is this regulation that permits statins and other cholesterol drugs to work so effectively.[4]

The majority of our cells make the cholesterol they need. The liver, however, is an especially efficient cholesterol factory, packaging much of its cholesterol into lipoproteins that can be delivered to cells throughout the body, providing a supplement to what each cell can make on its own. This supplement is especially important to the areas of the body that utilize a lot of cholesterol—like the testes in men and the ovaries in women, where the sex hormones are created.

Why do I bother to explain that the body makes its own cholesterol? Because I can't tell you how many patients look exasperated when I tell them they have high cholesterol. "Dr. Kennedy, I eat salads, and lots of fruits and vegetables. How can I have high cholesterol?" They seem both relieved and surprised to learn that their bodies manufacture their own cholesterol.

Diet comes into play because your blood cholesterol is determined by the following formula: How much your body makes + how much you take in from food = how much your body uses up or excretes. High cholesterol can result from a problem in any of the variables in that equation, including environmental, genetic and physiological factors. I had a patient a few years back that didn't excrete cholesterol in her bile efficiently. My patient Anne had familial combined hyperlipidemia, a genetic disease.

Here's the other thing you need to know about cholesterol and your diet. Your body will make cholesterol from any food—even a cholesterol-free food—as long as the food contains carbon—which carbohydrates, fats, and proteins all do. Carbon provides the body with the building blocks needed to make its own cholesterol. This may put a damper on the dietary ambitions of advocates of high saturated fat diets such as Atkins or the Paleo Diet, but it's true.

DIET: THE OTHER CHOLESTEROL SOURCE

For most people—especially those with high cholesterol—the liver and other cells aren't the body's only sources of cholesterol. Most of us are aware that the typical high-fat American diet also is loaded with cholesterol. But how does the cholesterol from chicken fingers and French fries eventually make its way to your arteries?

Cholesterol is a bad swimmer. It can't travel by its lonesome through our bloodstream. So it has to combine with certain proteins, which pick up the cholesterol and transport it to different parts of the body. Together, cholesterol and protein form a lipoprotein together.

Most cholesterol formed this way is LDL cholesterol, and this is the kind that's most likely to clog the blood vessels. Triglycerides and saturated fats are the first things to skyrocket after eating, especially a fatty meal. Why does LDL go up after a fatty meal but HDL, which counteracts effects of LDL by carrying it away from plaque jobsites, does not? Turns out, these fatty meals also release a lot of VLDL (very low density lipoprotein), the building blocks of LDL. The lipid core of the plaques that clog our arteries are filled with LDL.

IS EVEN A LITTLE CHOLESTEROL TOO MUCH?

The answer is "yes," if you happen to be Dr. T. Colin Campbell, the Jacob Gould Schurman Professor Emeritus of Nutritional Biochemistry at Cornell University, and author of the controversial *China Study.* "Eating foods that contain any cholesterol above 0 mg is unhealthy," said Dr. Campbell in the *China Study*, which was co-authored by his son. Controversial from the moment it was fresh off the presses, the *China Study*, his groundbreaking book that focused on the relationship between animal products consumption (including dairy) and a variety of chronic illnesses, such as coronary heart disease, diabetes, and cancer. Dr. Campbell's assertion that "any cholesterol above 0 mg is unhealthy," is drawn from a broad—and selective—pool of research. Yet, his NIH funded study, which found that while chemical carcinogens may initiate the cancer process, dietary promoters and anti-factor promoters control the promotion of cancer growth. Ultimately, nutritional factors, not chemical carcinogens, are the deciding factors in the development of cancer. As Dr. Campbell himself concluded, "Nutrients from animal-based foods increased tumor development while nutrients from plant-based foods decreased tumor development."

What can be learned from the *China Study* and Dr. Campbell's highly controversial conclusions about the causal relationship between dietary fat and the development of many chronic diseases?

Take Dr. Campbell assertion that "high-fat, high-protein, animal-based foods promote diabetes," while "high-fiber, whole, plant-based

(continues)

(continued)

foods protect against diabetes."[5] On the surface, it sounds logical since animal-based products contain more saturated fat than plant-based foods (notable exceptions include coconut, coconut oil, palm oil and palm kernel oil (often called tropical oils), and cocoa butter). But here's where things don't always add up. At one point, Dr. Campbell asserts, "plasma cholesterol...is positively associated with most cancer mortality rates. Plasma cholesterol is positively associated with animal protein intake and inversely associated with plant protein intake." High cholesterol is certainly associated with various cancers (the first genetic link between high cholesterol and cancer was discovered in 2012), and there's certainly less cholesterol in plant protein. No argument there. But when animal protein intake is correlated directly with cancer, there are as many negative as positive correlations, and none of the positive associations that I could find reaches what could be deemed a "statistically significant" threshold.

Dr. Campbell also engages in a lengthy discussion about casein, a milk protein that he believes causes cancer. Casein, he suggests, is associated with cancer when given in isolation—meaning independent of other milk proteins—to lab animals. The effects of casein—particularly isolated casein that's separated from other dairy components that work synergistically—can't be generalized to all forms of milk protein, much less all forms of animal protein. There are studies showing that whey, the other major milk protein, consistently suppresses tumor growth rather than promoting it, likely due to its ability to raise glutathione levels.[6,7]

Certainly, Dr. Campbell was well intentioned in his efforts. And as a whole, a plant-based diet is better and healthier, both for us and for our planet. I wouldn't argue otherwise. But the effect of animal-based protein is a complex issue, and conclusions can't be reached from epidemiologic data alone. How many of Dr. Campbell's research subjects were obese? Did their environment contribute to their health problems? How

(continues)

(continued)

physically active were they? Any researcher can approach a problem with preconceptions that allow him to see only what he wants to see.

As a cardiologist and scientist, I base nearly all of my medical decisions on clinical evidence. Of course, *The Heart Health Bible* is a prevention-based book and thus many of my recommendations fall outside the scope of evidence-based medicine. In fact, only an estimated 30 percent of doctors regularly follow evidence-based guidelines for treatment. "Trust your gut," is big part of allopathic medical practice. Still, I have to adhere to certain rules. I can't go off half-cocked. The hospital where I'm the director of preventive cardiology grades my diagnoses on the medications I prescribe. It's unfortunate but that's the way the system works. In reviewing my work, hospital administrators might see that I prescribe medications for CAD 85 percent of the time. But they will want to know why I don't prescribe medications 100 percent of time. Hospitals are worried about liability (who isn't these days?) and I don't want to subject myself to unnecessary criticism.

If I dissect an artery that caused a fatal heart attack, I will find in every instance that cholesterol was part of the plaque that caused the blockage. This plaque consists of a fibrous cap, smooth muscle, calcium, and a lipid core. That lipid core contains cholesterol. Every heart attack is caused when plaque ruptures and our body forms a clot, which causes the blockage. Cholesterol always is part of the plaque! Cholesterol is what makes the plaque vulnerable to a rupture.

Dietary cholesterol affects the progression of atherosclerosis. This is a scientific fact. It's not in dispute. The question is whether we can block that cholesterol with medication or through diet. In my estimation, we still don't have a great answer to this question.

DOES STRESS REALLY RAISE YOUR CHOLESTEROL LEVEL?

How bad is stress?

Stress can increase your heart rate, weaken your body's defenses, and increase certain inflammatory markers. We know this. But can stress also raise your cholesterol? It's a controversial subject, but one that appears to have legs, at least for some people, since there's now some evidence showing that how we react to prolonged stress directly impacts our lipid levels.

How we react to stress and whether this reaction can increase cholesterol and heighten future cardiovascular risk is an open question. We all respond differently to the everyday life challenges. People who respond poorly to stress have much higher levels of cholesterol, specifically LDL, than others who seem to cope better.

It's though that acute stress response, the classic "fight or flight" response, may raise fasting serum lipids. There are three reasons why this may be the case say the researchers. Stress may goad our bodies into producing more fatty acids and glucose—our "metabolic fuels." To do this, the liver produces and secretes additional LDL. Stress may interfere with lipid metabolism. A third possibility is that stress sets off known inflammatory processes such as the production of C-Reactive protein and Interlukin 6, both of which that are known to increase lipid production.

Why is the cholesterol/stress connection important? Simply, stress is a known heart disease risk factor that's in our power to do something about. I tell my patients you can't control your environment; you can't even control your effort. But you can always control your reactions. And that could make all the difference.[8]

WHAT YOU NEED TO KNOW

Patients with high cholesterol want to get better. But I'm also seeing an increasing number who want to know why they have a problem to begin with. I think the knowledge of the two goes hand in hand. Knowing how cholesterol is made in the body and how cholesterol is absorbed from food is the foundation for understanding how a great eating plan like my *5 for 1 Diet,* and, when necessary, cholesterol-lowering drugs are effective.

USING YOUR H-E-A-R-T

If you've been keeping an eye on your cholesterol levels, there's something else you might need to monitor: your triglycerides. As we learned in this chapter, triglycerides are part of our total cholesterol and the first fats to become elevated when we gain weight. They make up part of our total cholesterol and although not as harmful as low HDL and high LDL, triglycerides are also associated with increased cardiovascular risk. Having a high level of triglycerides can increase your risk of heart disease. However, the same lifestyle choices that promote overall health can help lower your triglycerides, too. This is why I tell my patients to "tackle their triglycerides." Following these rules will help your other cholesterol numbers as well.

MY FAVORITE PLANT FOODS

Here's a quick quiz: How do you know if a food is high in saturated fat? Take bacon as an obvious but still compelling example. Bacon grease is solid at room temperature, a sign that it's high in saturated fat because it prompts your body to make cholesterol. The big contributors of saturated fat in your diet are meats, dairy products, and eggs. Though there is some controversy surrounding this subject, it's my firm belief that the more you replace these products with plant-based foods, the better off you'll be.[9]

From my perspective, fish is a mixed bag. Fish fat contains omega-3 fats, also called "good fats," which are healthier in some ways that other animal fats. However, 70 to 85 percent of fish fat doesn't contain omega-3 fatty acids. It is a mixture of plain old saturated fat and various other fats that offer no tangible health benefits.

High cholesterol increases your risk of heart disease and heart attacks. This is an indisputable scientific fact. You can reduce cholesterol with medications, and there some people who may need to or even prefer this route. But if you'd rather try an alternate route to reduce your cholesterol, try these healthy lifestyle changes. If you're already taking medications, these changes will improve their cholesterol-lowering effect.

Lose weight

Carrying even just a few extra pounds contributes to high cholesterol. *Losing just 5 to 10 percent of your body weight can help significantly reduce cholesterol levels.* Start by making an honest, thorough look at your eating habits and daily routine. What are your biggest challenges? What foods are your biggest triggers? Do you eat even when you're not hungry? Can you develop strategies that will not only help you lose weight, but also keep the weight off?

For example, if you're an emotional eater—you eat when you're depressed, bored, or frustrated—consider a behavior that might deflect those feelings such as walking, knitting, or calling a friend. You can also try Listerine breath strips, which is a favorite strategy of renowned diet doctor Stephen Gullo, who has found that they are immediately effective at killing appetite. If you buy your lunch at a deli or fast food restaurant for lunch every day, try packing a healthier alternative at home. If you're traveling or don't have time to prepare lunch, most fast food chains offer low-calorie, heart-healthy alternatives. If you're sitting in front of the television, which encourages mindless eating behavior, try munching on carrot sticks instead of potato chips as you watch. Again taking a page from Dr. Gullo, whatever method you find works best for you and your lifestyle, remember that strategy and not willpower is the key to lasting weight loss.

And look for ways to "energize" for a healthy heart by incorporating more activity into your daily routine, such as using the stairs instead of taking the elevator. Take stock of what you currently eat and your physical activity level and slowly work in changes.

Eat Heart-Healthy Foods

Even if you have years of unhealthy eating under your belt, making just one or two small changes in your diet can reduce cholesterol and improve your heart health. A full selection of heart-healthy alternatives, including many great tasting gourmet recipes prepared by leading chefs, can be found in Chapter 9.

Choose Healthier Fats

Saturated fats, found in red meat and dairy products, raise your total cholesterol and low-density lipoprotein (LDL) cholesterol. Putting aside arguments that we should eat like our Paleolithic ancestors, many of whom died of diseases we now take for granted and none of whom ate bacon for breakfast, to my knowledge, you should get fewer than 7 percent of your daily calories from saturated fat. As an alternative, choose leaner cuts of meat, low-fat dairy, and monounsaturated fats, the sort found in olive, peanut, and canola oils.

Banish Trans Fats

Trans fat is a manmade fat that was created to protect us from butter. The problem is that it behaves worse than butter in our bodies. A process known as hydrogenation, in which vegetable oils are converted to solid fats by adding hydrogen atoms, creates trans fats.

This process adds shelf life and stabilizes the flavor of foods. Trans fatty acids are found naturally in small quantities in some foods including beef, pork, lamb, butter, and milk, but most trans fatty acids in the diet come from hydrogenated foods. When it comes to eating for a healthy heart, few things are worse than trans fats. The list of their crimes include increasing total cholesterol and LDL cholesterol, reducing HDL cholesterol, and interfering with the body's use of Omega-3 fatty acids, which are beneficial to our heart.

Limit Cholesterol in Your Food

Aim for no more than 300 milligrams (mg) of cholesterol a day— less than 200 mg if you have heart disease or diabetes. The most concentrated sources of cholesterol include organ meats, egg yolks and whole milk products. Use lean cuts of meat, egg substitutes and skim milk instead.

Select Whole Grains

Various nutrients found in whole grains promote heart health. Choose whole-grain breads, whole-wheat pasta, whole-wheat flour and brown rice.

Stock Up On Fruits And Vegetables

Fruits and vegetables are rich in dietary fiber, which can help lower cholesterol. Snack on seasonal fruits. Experiment with veggie-based casseroles, soups, and stir-fries. If you prefer dried fruit to fresh fruit limit yourself to no more than a handful (about an ounce or two). People tend to think of dried fruit as a healthy alternative to traditional snack foods. But dried fruit tends to have more calories than does fresh fruit. And since it's been cut into smaller pieces and "dried," people tend to lose track of how much they're eating and can quickly end up consuming more calories than they intended.

Eat Foods Rich In Omega-3 Fatty Acids

Omega-3 fatty acids can help lower your LDL ("bad") cholesterol. Some types of fish—such as salmon, mackerel, and herring—are rich in omega-3 fatty acids. Other good sources of omega-3 fatty acids include walnuts, almonds and ground flaxseeds.

Exercise Most Days of the Week

Whether you're overweight or not, exercise has been shown to reduce cholesterol. Even better, moderate physical activity can help raise high-density lipoprotein (HDL) cholesterol. If you don't exercise regularly, try working up to thirty minutes of exercise a day at least five to six days a week. Remember that adding physical activity, even in ten-minute intervals several times a day, can help you begin to lose weight. Just be sure that you can keep up the changes you decide to make. And always check with your healthcare provider before starting any exercise program, especially if you have an existing health condition.

Consider:

Taking a brisk daily walk during your lunch hour
Riding your bike to work
Swimming laps
Playing a favorite sport

To stay motivated, find an exercise buddy or join an exercise group. Exercising with a friend helps make you accountable. Who wants to be the person who didn't show up? And remember, any activity is helpful. Even taking the stairs instead of the elevator or doing a few sit-ups while watching television can make a difference.

If You Smoke, Stop. Period!

Quitting may improve your HDL cholesterol level. And the benefits don't end there. Just twenty minutes after quitting, your blood pressure decreases. Within twenty-four hours, your risk of a heart attack decreases. Within one year, your risk of heart disease is half that of a smoker. Within fifteen years, your risk of heart disease is similar to someone who never smoked.

Drink Alcohol Sparingly or Avoid Altogether

Moderate use of alcohol has been linked with higher levels of HDL cholesterol. But drinking too much alcohol can lead to serious health problems as well, including high blood pressure, heart failure, and stroke. And when it comes to alcohol, most people aren't given to moderation but to excess. Remember that alcohol has a disinhibiting effect, meaning that if you drink, especially on an empty stomach, you may end consuming a lot of extra calories. Also, many alcoholic fruit drinks like a pina coladas have as many calories as a dinner entrée. For healthy adults, I often recommend one drink a day for women of all ages and men older than age sixty-five, and up to two drinks a day for men age sixty-five and younger. But just remember that just one drink a day can cost you more than 36,000 calories annually! So if you don't drink, don't start. The limited benefits aren't enough to recommend alcohol for anyone who doesn't already drink.

If lifestyle changes aren't enough . . .

Sometimes healthy lifestyle changes aren't enough to lower cholesterol levels. Make sure the changes you choose to make are ones that you can continue, and don't be disappointed if you don't see results immediately. If your doctor recommends medication to help lower your cholesterol, take it as prescribed, but continue your lifestyle changes.

Tackling triglycerides requires adopting some or all of these healthy lifestyle choices. Write them down and start incorporating them into your daily routine today.

THE BOTTOM LINE: RECOMMENDATIONS FOR FAT INTAKE

Although the different types of fat have a varied—and admittedly confusing—effect on health and disease, the basic message is simple: Out with the bad, in with the good. You can do this by choosing foods with healthy fats, limiting foods that are high in saturated fat, and avoiding trans-fat. Here's how to make it happen:

Eliminate trans fats from partially hydrogenated oils. Food labels should say "0" (zero) on the line for trans-fat; also scan the ingredient list to make sure it does not contain partially hydrogenated oils (food labeling laws allow food makers to have up to 0.5 grams of trans fat in a product but still list "0" on the line for trans fats). Fortunately, most food manufacturers have removed trans fats from their products. In restaurants, steer clear of fried foods, biscuits, and other baked goods, unless you know that the restaurant has eliminated trans-fat (many already have).

Limit your intake of saturated fats by cutting back on red meat and full-fat dairy foods. Try replacing red meat with beans, nuts, poultry, and fish whenever possible, and switching from whole milk and other full-fat dairy foods to lower fat versions, or just eating smaller amounts of full-fat dairy products, such as cheese. Don't replace red meat with refined carbohydrates (white bread, white rice, potatoes, and the like).

In place of butter, use liquid vegetable oils rich in polyunsaturated and monounsaturated fats, in cooking and at the table. Olive oil, canola oil, sunflower oil, safflower oil, corn oil, peanut oil, and the like are great sources of healthy fat.

Eat one or more good sources of omega-3 fats every day. Fish, walnuts, canola or soybean oil, ground flax seeds or flaxseed oil are excellent sources of omega-3 fats.

As you choose foods with healthy fat, and limit the amount of trans and saturated fats in your diet, keep in mind that replacing saturated fat with refined carbohydrates will not protect you against heart disease and may even raise your risk. But there is solid proof that replacing saturated fat with unsaturated fats will help lower your heart disease risk.

ONE FINAL THOUGHT

As you follow the recommendations above for tackling triglycerides and controlling your cholesterol, remember that your "numbers" are only part of the equation. H-E-A-R-T doesn't just measure your cholesterol levels. More important, use it as a measure of the behaviors that led to your high cholesterol since in 90 percent of cases, it's what we do and think that contributes to our problems.

CHAPTER 9

Diet: Eat for 5, Dine for 1

"Cut all fat from your diet." "Don't eat too much saturated fat." "Add more fruits and vegetables." "Eat this, not that." "But hold the presses: 50% of your diet *should* consist of saturated fat?"

Confused? You're not alone. What is the optimal heart-healthy diet? Ask five experts and you'll get five different answers. It's confusing, especially for those inundated with a plethora of well-intentioned but often misguided advice. However, here's a little morsel that is not in dispute: Almost 70 percent of adult Americans are overweight or obese. If current trends continue, it's estimated that 165 million Americans will be obese by 2030. Healthy eating, in particular, is the Achilles' heel of heart smart aspirations. Why? It's a sad truth that in a world of thousands upon thousands of diet programs, few, if any, produce lasting weight loss. As Dr. James A. Levine, a leading endocrinologist at the prestigious Mayo Clinic observed in a recent *New York Times* article, "We really haven't come up with one good weight-loss solution. If we had, everyone would be using it." In this chapter, I've created a new blueprint for heart-healthy eating, one so powerful that it will enable people who suffer with coronary heart disease, high cholesterol, obesity and/or high blood pressure to reduce or perhaps even eliminate their dependence on medications and avoid costly and invasive surgical procedures.

FINDING THE MOTIVATION TO CHANGE: CLARK'S STORY

For Clark, a 27-year-old Internet entrepreneur and angel investor, things started early, as they do for most people with weight problems. Growing up, everything seemed to revolve around eating. At family celebrations there was food. When Clark came home from school, his mother handed him a snack. When he received a great report card, he got ice cream or cupcakes; when he was feeling down or sad, it was "eat something, you'll feel better"; when he was bored or didn't have anything to do, he ate. By the time Clark reached age 12, he was 5' 3" and 200 pounds.

Despite a long family history of heart disease, diabetes, and stroke, Clark's parents did not seem too concerned with their son's ballooning weight. After all, "he's just a boy," his mom rationalized. "No cause for alarm." Compounding matters was that everyone in Clark's family, from his parents to his youngest sibling, was overweight or obese. "Not a skinny one in the bunch," Clark's grandmother was fond of saying. But in Clark's family, the emperors all were wearing no clothes. They blithely shared in the collective ignorance of an obvious fact—they were all fat, and dangerously so. Family weight problems were the proverbial 5,000-pound elephant that everyone chose to ignore.

By the time he finished graduate school, Clark was experiencing intermittent mild chest pains, and he was tired and fatigued all the time. These symptoms continued on and off for two more years, until Clark was diagnosed with high blood pressure, unstable angina and borderline diabetes following a routine office visit.

Clark's physician suggested he consult with me. Though he'd been overweight his whole life and was consistently besieged by doctor after doctor to lose weight, Clark was shocked to learn that he was "morbidly obese," as I told him in no uncertain terms after our first consult. "Clark you're 5'8" and you weigh 300 pounds. You have a BMI of 45.6 (anything over 30 is considered obese). You fall under the category of 'morbidly obese'."

We needed a plan of action, fast. Either Clark was going to do something about his weight, or the next time I saw him it would be for angioplasty. As we discussed options for losing weight, I even thought of referring Clark to my colleague Jeremy Korman, perhaps our country's leading bariatric surgeon and one of my favorite people. However, after talking to Clark for nearly an hour, it dawned on me that he didn't have a weight problem. What do I mean by that? After all, Clark was tipping the scales at 300. It was obvious to anyone that Clark's weight was leading him down the path to a lifetime's worth of health problems, not the least of which was an increased risk of heart attack or even cardiac arrest. What I mean is that Clark's weight was a symptom—a symptom of being out of control with food. As I shared my thoughts with Clark, he abruptly stopped our conversation. "Look, Dr. Kennedy, I know that I have a weight problem but that has nothing to do with my head. I just need to lose a few pounds. Then I'll be fine."

In fact, Clark wouldn't be fine. For one, many of these foods he craved—pizza and potato chips just to name two—and "couldn't do without," were literally rewiring his brain and tampering with its reward system, upping the satisfaction threshold to such a degree that too much would never be enough.

The problem vexing Clark had little to do with his food choices and everything to do with his head. Unless Clark changed his fundamental thoughts and feelings about food, particularly the early childhood programming that was at the root of his weight problems, he would see me again, which not coincidentally happened just a week later when Clark was wheeled into the emergency room complaining of tightness and pain in his chest, jaw, and left arm. Clark also was short of breath and shared that he was experiencing "overwhelming anxiety and an impending feeling of doom." Bottom line: Clark was having a heart attack.

With a heart attack, heart tissue loses oxygen and dies so blood flow has to be restored in a hurry. Clark was taken to the hospital's catheterization laboratory, where I performed emergency coronary angioplasty and put in a stent to open two blocked coronary arteries. I simultaneously performed a coronary angioplasty at the same time as a coronary catheterization to locate the blocked arteries.

Sitting in Clark's hospital room the following day it was clear that he felt ashamed. "I feel bad now that I didn't listen to you, Dr. Kennedy." I assured Clark that his arteries were 80% occluded and his heart disease so advanced that surgery was inevitable. My question to Clark was where do we go from here? "I know I have to eat less and exercise more," said Clark, adding that he was committed to adopting a "heart-healthy eating plan." While all of this sounded good, I told Clark that based on what I knew about his background, upbringing, and issues surrounding food making a few cosmetic changes to his diet, or even adopting a heart-healthy eating plan, would just be icing on the cake. Until Clark changed the way he thought about food and finally overcame the early childhood programming that had led him to gain weight again and again, he wouldn't make lasting changes to weight, waistline and overall health. "Clark, it was Einstein who said, 'We cannot solve our problems with the same *thinking* we used when we created them.' This is what you're trying to do. This is why you're never going to succeed at losing weight and more importantly, keep it off."

Clark seemed taken aback by my comments. *But as we discussed things further, he realized that the root of his weight problems wasn't the food but the way he thought about food.* Dieters change their eating habits to lose weight. But once they reach their target goal most return to same behavior patterns that led them to gain weight in the first place. Perhaps this is why the average American dieter makes up to 5 weight-loss attempts a year.

A WEIGHTY PROBLEM THAT KEEPS GETTING BIGGER

You don't have to be a rocket scientist to realize that we're in the throes of a weight epidemic in this country. Forget all the stories you read or statistics you hear on the evening news. Want proof? Just visit your local supermarket. You'll see cautionary tales perusing the aisles, filling their carts with every high calorie, non-nutritive food imaginable. At the checkout line, tabloid headlines scream about a certain celebrity who regained and then some the eighty pounds she lost after following a popular diet program. Oprah Winfrey has literally redefined the term "yo-yo dieting." Not only is our never-ending battle with the bulge demoralizing, but also the gain-lose-gain cycle has been linked to potentially life-threatening conditions such as high blood pressure, high cholesterol, diabetes, depression, heart disease, and cancer.

But if you count up the casualties of the weight war, celebrities represent only the very tip of the proverbial diet iceberg. Look around. Really big bodies are everywhere. At a majority of this country's restaurants, the typical entrée falls way outside the USDA recommendations for salt, fat and saturated fat. Serving sizes have more than doubled in the last twenty years both inside and outside the home. Compounding the problem is that most of us are plate cleaners. When was the last time you went to a fine restaurant and left half your meal on the plate? Whether you want a lot of food or not, the more you're served, the more you eat.[1]

Not only are we eating too much, but we're also struggling to lose weight and more important, keep it off. A study published a few years ago in the venerable *New England Journal of Medicine* reported that two-thirds of dieters regain all the weight they lose within a year, and more than 95% gain it all back within five years.[2] After analyzing thirty-one long-term diet studies, UCLA researchers found that about two-thirds of dieters regained more weight within four or five years than they initially lost.[3]

Imagine if I told you that almost 70 percent of the population had cancer, AIDS or even worse, ALS. What would you do? How would react to that news? It would be cause for a national emergency. But when it comes to weight, few of us seem to bat an eyelash when I share that almost 70 percent—68.8 percent to be exact—of adult Americans are overweight or obese. For all the talk about the overweight/obesity epidemic becoming a front and center topic of conversation, little is being done to solve the problem. Indeed, if trends continue, the 68.8 percent is expected to jump to 75 percent by 2020 and 80 percent by 2030.[4]

But why does it matter that we have a nationwide weight problem? If some guy at the table next to you wants to stuff himself to capacity with French fries and milk shakes, why is that any of your business? It's a free country after all. But you should care. We should all be deeply concerned. This country's weight crisis imperils our physical, economic, and social well being. If you're overweight, you're statistically at greater risk for developing type 2 diabetes, hypertension, heart disease, stroke, osteoarthritis, and certain cancers. Is it any wonder that type 2 diabetes has risen a staggering 76 percent in the last twenty years despite the availability of insulin analogs (an altered form of insulin that's unlike any occurring in nature, but still available to the human body for performing the same action as human insulin in terms of glycemic control)?[5] Even a small amount of excess weight, accumulated slowly at the rate of one to two pounds a year over many years, can lead to type 2 diabetes.

Not only is obesity a threat to our bottoms, it's also a threat to our nation's bottom line. The total economic cost of overweight and obesity in the U.S. and Canada now exceeds $300 billion per year (90 percent of which is attributable to the U.S.). The staggering overweight and obesity numbers are caused by an increased need for medical care, and loss of economic productivity resulting from excess mortality and disability, the study found. Slicing up the $270 billion bill in this country, obesity cost the U.S. economy $198 billion and overweight cost $72 billion in 2009. Of this $270 billion, medical care caused by overweight and obesity came in at $127 billion. Simply put, the fat epidemic is an extraordinary economic burden on society.[6]

And there are other, less obvious costs that go far beyond dollars and cents. As much as it pains me to say and as unfair as it may be, many overweight and obese are societal outcasts. Overweight and obese people are less likely to be given jobs, they're waited on more slowly in stores and restaurants, they're less likely to be given apartments, and they're even less likely to be college educated.[7]

When it comes to weight problems, all communities aren't affected equally. It's a sad fact that obesity rates are higher in some ethnic communities and in lower-income states. The trends are so extreme that they are attracting the attention of health officials and lawmakers.

Obesity among children is also rising, and it's a real threat that may have lasting health consequences. From my own practice of preventive and interventional cardiology, I've been seeing far too many overweight and obese children who are at risk for a host of health problems if things don't change, quickly. And like their adults counterparts, minority and low-income children are disproportionately affected by obesity. Black and Latino children are more likely to be at risk for being overweight and obese than White children. It's estimated that 20 percent of Black children ages 2 to 19 are obese, compared with approximately 14 percent of White children. Black and Latino children are more likely to be diagnosed with type 2 diabetes, a disease strongly associated with being overweight and obese. Socioeconomic status factors into the equation, as almost 45 percent of overweight or obese children ages 10 to 17 are poor.[8]

WHY DO WE OVEREAT?

It's an interesting question with a not so obvious answer. Some experts maintain that at the level of our genes, we're programmed to eat as much as we can to survive and then store the extra as fat for future use. At first glance, this notion seems far-fetched. Is it really possible after almost 300,000 years of evolution that our brains still cling to the Darwinian desire for high calorie, high fat foods? Clearly, our Paleolithic ancestors, out of necessity, sought out calorie rich goodies. They couldn't pop by the local twenty-four-hour mini-mart when hunger hit. High calorie foods were certainly scarce. Thus, the comparatively primitive brains of our forbearers may have developed neural pathways that heightened their desire for high calories foods. Indeed, we now know from neuroimaging studies that food floods our brains with dopamine, a neurotransmitter that controls the brain's reward and pleasure centers, enabling us to both see rewards and to then take action to fulfill them. If we receive enough positive reinforcement from food—think about how great it feels to munch on a handful of potato chips or eat a slice of chocolate cake—then we start seeking out anything—people, places, stores—we associate with that food.

This heightened biological sensitivity may explain why certain foods trigger cravings, increase appetite, and cause us to fall off the heart-healthy food wagon. Even the most obdurate dieter may find it impossible to withstand the powerful biological forces that cause us to seek out and obtain calorie-rich treats. Perhaps this is what led Nora Volkow, M.D., Director of Programming at the National Institute on Drug Abuse (NIDA) at the National Institutes of Health, to exclaim, "We are programmed to pig out on calories."

The larger issue, quite literally, is that we live in a twenty-four-hour food environment, where any calorie-dense, sugar-laden and/or fatty food is available around every corner. Food isn't scarce. It's plentiful. Thus, these neural pathways may no longer be in our best interest.

And it's not just biology that shapes our food destiny. Experiences, attitudes, and cultural conditioning dramatically affect our food preferences and desires. From advertising billboards to pop up banner ads and everything in between, a never-ending stream of external cues trigger us to eat and even orient us in the direction of certain foods. Look around. We're drowning in an ocean of food stores, fast food chains, food courts, twenty-four-hour-a-day diners, and all you can eat buffets. With profit margins on gasoline amounting to just a few cents on the dollar, almost every gas station's "real bread and butter is really bread and butter," as a recent report by NBC News pointed out. The food items sold at gas station convenience stores generate much higher profits than gas.[9]

Today, it's all but impossible to escape the slick ads, commercials, and infomercials that reinforce the belief that food is indispensable to a good life. Advertisers spend billions on brightly colored, shiny, cleverly worded packaging that is specifically designed to get us to buy and over consume. Coupled with powerful cultural and biological programming and surrounded by messages that food is the ultimate reward, is it any surprise that majority of citizens in this country are overweight or obese?

METABOLIC MATHEMATICS

Small weight fluctuations are normal. If you go out for a long run, or on the opposite end, enjoy a celebratory meal, you'll likely see a few pounds come or go. This happens to all of us. On the other hand, weight cycling, more commonly known as "yo-yo dieting," is an unhealthy behavior marked by a significant increase or decrease of body weight—ten pounds or more—that occurs over and over again.

Though weight cycling is known to be bad for our health, Kelly Brownell, PhD., newly appointed director of Duke University's Sanford School of Public Policy, and the man credited with coining the expression "yo-yo dieting," says the matter may not be entirely under our control. Dr. Brownell speculates that every time we diet, our bodies perceive the weight loss as a threat to their survival. "[The body] might not know the difference between Atkins and famine," he told *Women's Health online*. Moreover, says Dr. Brownell, weight cycling probably changes our physiology, meaning the more diets we try, the harder it is to lose weight.[10] Our bodies don't like change and they may respond to each new diet by increasing the production of a hunger hormone called ghrelin while decreasing production of leptin, a satiety hormone. Bottom line: With every diet, we feel hungrier and less satisfied. (Obesity, it's worth noting, scrambles both hormones and their signals.) Is it any wonder a majority of this country's 108 million dieters keep falling off the wagon?

Other studies point out that the never-ending cycle of losing and regaining weight wreaks havoc with our metabolism. Restrictive diets that result in rapid weight loss might be great if you want to fit into a new black dress or are scrambling to lose weight before beach season kicks into high bear. But they could also have the undesired effect of causing you to lose more muscle than fat. Problems arise if you gain back the weight, which the majority of dieters do, since it might come back as fat, which is ten times less metabolically active than muscle. This nasty cycle effectively lowers your metabolism, compounding the challenge of losing weight. Thus, the more times you diet, the harder it will be for you to lose weight. And with an average of five weight loss attempts a year, most dieters will find in no time that their metabolism has slowed to a snail's pace.

Weight cycling isn't just a physical phenomenon; emotional triggers play a huge role, too. Dieters who eat in response to stress, boredom, depression, or loneliness — as opposed to external events like happy hour, tailgating before a football game, or a celebratory meal also struggle to keep weight off.

PORTION DISTORTION

While we're slowing down our metabolism with repeated attempts at dieting, we're also increasing our portion sizes, to which our waist-lines have responded accordingly. Certainly, the overweight/obesity epidemic can't be laid squarely at the feet of larger portion sizes, but big quantities of cheap food may have distorted our perceptions of what a typical meal is supposed to look like, while conditioning us to expect the biggest bang for our buck.

How much have portion sizes grown? Twenty years ago, two slices of pizza averaged 500 calories. Today, those same slices weigh in at 850 calories. Those extra 350 calories, if eaten just three times a month, would put on three extra pounds a year, or 60 pounds in the next two decades. Twenty years ago, a 16-oz coffee with milk and sugar would cost you 90 calories. Today, a Grande Café Mocha with whip cream made from 2% milk totals 330 calories. The extra 240 calories consumed four times a week would add nearly four pounds a year or 80 pounds after 20 years. But who wants a plain old 8-oz cup of coffee in a nondescript Styrofoam cup? Today, it's not unusual to see 32-ounce coffee cups, four times the size they used to be. Several popular coffees have as many calories as a full meal. There are many more examples. Move popcorn, a dubious choice for many dieters to begin with, registered at 270 calories for 5 cups 20 years ago. Now, a tub of popcorn clocks in at 630.[11] How is it possible that anyone could eat this much popcorn? For one, I've found—and studies bear this out—that people will consume more if they're given large containers, even if they're not that hungry!

Across the board, portion sizes have escalated. At fast food chains, portion sizes are two to five times larger than when first introduced. The 160-calorie, single serving can of Coke seems like an anachronism in the face of a 20-ounce plastic bottle, which contains 2.5 servings and comes in at 240 calories.[12] These larger sizes make it nearly impossible for people to manage how much they're taking in.

DO YOU KNOW YOUR PORTION SIZES?

Do you suffer from portion distortion? Take the National Heart, Lung, and Blood Institute's Portion Distortion Quiz.

1. A bagel 20 years ago was 3 inches in diameter and had 140 calories. How many calories do you think are in today's bagel?

   a. 150 calories
   b. 250 calories
   c. 350 calories

2. A cheeseburger 20 years ago had 333 calories. How many calories do you think are in today's cheeseburger?

   a. 590 calories
   b. 620 calories
   c. 700 calories

3. A 6.5-ounce portion of soda had 85 calories 20 years ago. How many calories do you think are in today's portion?

   a. 200 calories
   b. 250 calories
   c. 300 calories

4. 2.4 ounces of French fries 20 years ago had 210 calories. How many calories do you think are in today's portion?

   a. 590 calories
   b. 610 calories
   c. 650 calories

5. A portion of spaghetti and meatballs 20 years ago had 500 calories. How many calories do you think are in today's portion of spaghetti and meatballs?

   a. 600 calories
   b. 800 calories
   c. 1,025 calories

(continues)

(continued)

6. A cup of coffee with milk and sugar 20 years ago was 8 ounces and had 45 calories. How many calories do you think are in today's mocha coffee?

    a. 100 calories
    b. 350 calories
    c. 450 calories

7. A muffin 20 years ago was 1.5 ounces and had 210 calories. How many calories do you think are in a muffin today?

    a. 320 calories
    b. 400 calories
    c. 500 calories

8. Two slices of pepperoni pizza 20 years ago had 500 calories. How many calories do you think are in today's large pizza slices?

    a. 850 calories
    b. 1,000 calories
    c. 1,200 calories

9. A chicken Caesar salad had 390 calories 20 years ago. How many calories do you think are in today's chicken Caesar salad?

    a. 520 calories
    b. 650 calories
    c. 790 calories

10. A box of popcorn had 270 calories 20 years ago. How many calories do you think are in today's tub of popcorn?

    a. 520 calories
    b. 630 calories
    c. 820 calories

Thank you for taking the Portion Distortion Quiz. We hope it was fun and insightful. We also hope that next time you eat out, you will think twice about the food portions offered to you.

(continues)

(continued)

Answers

1. c. 350 calories for a 6-inch bagel. If you rake leaves for 50 minutes you'll burn the extra 210 calories.*

2. a. 590 calories. You'll need to lift weights for 1 hour and 30 minutes to burn the extra, approximately 250 calories.*

3. b. 250 calories for a 20-ounce soda. If you work in the garden for 35 minutes you will burn the extra 165 calories.**

4. b. 610 calories for a 6.9 ounce portion of French fries. If you walk leisurely for 1 hour and 10 minutes, you will burn the extra 400 calories.**

5. c. 1,025 calories for a portion consisting of 2 cups of pasta with sauce and 3 large meatballs. If you houseclean for 2 hours and 35 minutes, you will burn approximately 525 calories.*

6. b. 350 calories for a 16-ounce cup of coffee. If you walk approximately 1 hour and 20 minutes, you will burn the extra 310 calories.*

7. c. 500 calories for a 5-ounce muffin. If you vacuum for approximately 1 hour and 30 minutes you will burn the extra 310 calories.*

8. a. 850 calories for 2 large slices of pizza. If you play golf (while walking and carrying your clubs) for 1 hour, you will burn the extra 350 calories.**

9. c. 790 calories for a 3-cup portion. If you walk the dog for 1 hour and 20 minutes, you will burn the extra 400 calories.**

10. b. 630 calories for a tub of popcorn. If you do water aerobics for 1 hour and 15 minutes, you will burn the extra 360 calories.**

*Based on a 130-pound person
**Based on a 160-pound person

A 2004 study published in the journal *Appetite* found that as package size increased, so did consumption; subjects ate up to 37 percent more with the bigger bags.[13]

The containers we use to hold are larger food portions have jumped as well. Plates, bowls, and cup sizes have all shot up. In the last twenty years, the standard size of a dinner plate has increased from ten to twelve inches. A study in the venerable *American Journal of Preventive Medicine* found that people given larger bowls and spoons helped themselves to larger portions of ice cream and often ate the whole portion.[14]

YOUR BRAIN ON FOOD

The other problem stemming from larger portion sizes has everything to do with the foods we're supersizing. It's been obvious to me for the longest time that sweet, salty, crunchy, and fatty foods are appetite triggers. I don't ever remember seeing a patient who overate steamed broccoli or stewed tomatoes. Growing evidence has now demonstrated that certain foods mimic drugs of abuse in their effect on our brains, even leading to long-term changes in the two parts of the hypothalamus—the brain's command control for hunger and eating. One area, the Ventromedial Nuclei, gives a signal when to stop eating; the other, the Lateral hypothalamus, signals when it's time to start eating.

Some of the changes are so profound that they don't go away, even if we return to a normal diet. This is really no different than what happens after long-term drug abuse. The brain's reward circuitry changes to such an extent that it triggers cravings and promotes the seeking of that drug. In a study published in the journal *Neuroscience*, researchers followed rats that had learned to give themselves heroin by pressing a lever. When the scientists removed the heroin, the rats mostly stopped pressing the lever. But when the scientists took away the rat's food, the lever pressing ensued with a vengeance.

In fact, the rats pressed the lever hundreds of times. Sugar, as an example, is potentially addictive enough that it led rats in a separate study to seek it the way addicts seek drugs.[15]

With the cards clearly stacked against us, it's normal to wonder if we'd all just be better off ditching our diets, and just accept a few extra pounds. But with millions overweight or obese, we're not talking about just a few extra pounds. And the fallout from being overweight still far outweighs the risks of yo-yo dieting, especially where our hearts are concerned. The evidence is clear: There is an undeniable and powerful connection between being overweight or obese and having heart disease. The heart, truly the human body's hardest-working muscle, doesn't stop for bathroom breaks, lunch, or vacations. It spends every second of every day enthusiastically pumping blood to the farthest reaches of our bodies. The larger we become, the more our hearts have to pump and the harder they have to work to keep blood circulating.

Being overweight is such a problem that it literally changes in the structure and function of the heart. The more you weigh, the more blood you have flowing through your body. The heart has to work harder to pump the extra blood. It stretches and gets bigger. The heart muscle gets thicker. The thicker the heart muscle gets, the harder it is for it to squeeze and relax with each heartbeat. Over time, the heart may not be able to keep up with the extra load. You may then have heart failure.

So what exactly is the best way to jump on and more important, remain on the diet bandwagon? Despite the grim forecast, it's possible to change the conversation.

HEADFIRST

To begin, think less about the food on your plate, and more about the thoughts in your head. Even the most tempting donut is just a piece of food. It doesn't have a brain of its own. It can't outwit us. It's embodied only with the power we give it. The excess pounds millions of us carry around come less from the foods we choose than from our thoughts and feelings about those foods. The 100 or so calories in a handful of potato chips or 2 small chocolate chip cookies can't possibly account for 68 million overweight and obese adults, 400,000 deaths annually, an increased risk of heart disease, type 2 diabetes, and colon, breast, and endometrial cancer, and billions wasted in lost productivity. In fact, just a handful of potato chips shouldn't be a problem. But how many people do you know will only eat a handful of potato chips? It's not the number of calories in a handful of chips but how you behave in the face of those chips that's the issue.

PATIENCE IS A VIRTUE

Ten pounds in ten days sounds great but for most of us, it's neither realistic nor sustainable. You didn't gain the extra weight you're carrying around overnight. Reducing your weight by 10 percent over six months may not be as gratifying at ten in ten, but it's more realistic.

THINK LIFESTYLE

Most dieters lose at least some weight. Indeed, weight loss isn't the problem for the majority of this country's 108 million dieters. The problem is maintaining that weight loss. There's a reason why 95 percent of dieters eventually gain back all the weight they lose. All diets have a beginning, middle and end. Just look at two recent bestsellers "The 17-Day Diet" and "Lose 10 Pounds in 3 Days." The titles say it all. Diets, in and of themselves, are a temporary fix. Permanent weight loss and an end to cycle of yo-yo dieting is something much greater. It's a lifestyle.

ENERGIZE

Though studies show that exercise is better for maintenance than for weight loss, physical activity is useful because it gives structure and focus, no small consideration for anyone who feels out of control with their eating. Members of the National Weight Control Registry (an ongoing study of adults who have lost at least 30 pounds and kept it off for a year) cite exercise as a key strategy to help keep the pounds off. Just walking for thirty to sixty minutes at a pace of three to four miles per hour at least five days a week can slash your risk of heart disease by 40 percent.[16] If age or infirmity limits or even prohibits you from exercising, try ten to fifteen minutes of meditation, which has been shown to increase EEG coherence, blood flow to the brain, muscle relaxation, and decrease the production of stress hormones.

BANISH NEGATIVE THINKING

In a recent speech to the graduating class at Harvard, the author J. K. Rowling all but ignored any talk of her successes and chose instead to concentrate on her failures. As she told the audience, "...it is impossible to live without failing at something, unless you live so cautiously that you might as well not have lived at all—in which case, you fail by default." Nowhere is Rowling's sage advice more useful than in the world of dieting. One of the most important tips for losing weight and keeping it off is to remember that failing is normal. You will fail many times. They key is to learn from your failures so hopefully you gain more insight about what to do differently on the next go around.

THE 5 FOR 1 DIET

I think it is important to know what foods have been shown to be good for your heart and why. Dieting is perhaps the most common discussion topics in cardiology clinics. Always, we discuss the best way to eat to protect your heart. And dieting is important since it can have a significant impact on your long-term heart health. A recent study, published in the journal *Circulation*, shows just how beneficial a heart-healthy diet can be. In the study, researchers collected data on the amount of milk, vegetables, fruits, grains, fish, meat and poultry 31,000 participants with heart disease ate in the previous year. Over five years, 5,000 people had a heart attack or stroke. The results found that those who ate a heart-healthy diet reduced their risk of dying from heart disease by 35 percent.[17] Nice!

But what constitutes a "heart-healthy diet?" The list seems to change as often as the weather. The American Heart Association recommends that an adult eating 2,000 calories a day should have at least four-and-a-half cups of fruits and vegetables, eat fiber-rich whole grains and oily fish, and limit his or her sodium intake to less than 1,500 milligrams per day.

But multiple factors influence the development and progression of cardiovascular disease. And what I've noticed after hundreds of hours of conversations, that majority of the talk has centered around an overemphasis on foods to avoid rather than emphasis on heart-healthy foods to include. Avoid saturated fat, curb the simple carbs, and check your salt intake. The list goes on and on. Clearly, there is merit in eliminating a number of foods from our diet. But even people with just a marginal knowledge of nutrition probably know what foods to avoid. Honestly, is there anyone left in the country who thinks that French fries are a heart-healthy food? I'd prefer to emphasize the hundreds, if not thousands of delicious foods we should include in a heart-healthy diet.

What if I simplified things? Wouldn't it be great if all the information you needed was distilled into one place and organized in a way that allowed you to create fun, tasty gourmet recipes from ingredients that have all been proven to help you follow your H-E-A-R-T. It would be. That's why I created the 5 for 1 Diet. Learning about all the foods shown to heal your blood pressure, energize your heart, act on fat, reduce blood sugar, and tackle triglycerides is advantageous for all of us.

My recommendations for following the 5 for 1 Diet are simple. Every time you sit down to a meal or snack, I want you to hold up five fingers. You should eat for at least one if not all five of the five steps outlined in the HEART HEALTH BIBLE:

H — HEAL YOUR BLOOD PRESSURE
E — ENERGIZE YOUR HEART
A — ACT ON FAT
R — REDUCE BLOOD SUGAR
T — TACKLE TRIGYLCERIDES.

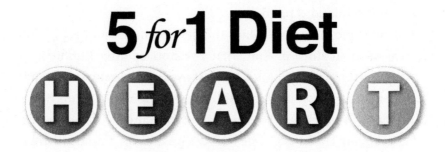

The following diet contains lists of foods that when eaten in appropriate portions can lower your risk of heart disease.

- Choose foods and nutrients from list **H** and lower your blood pressure.
- Choose foods and nutrients from list **E** and energize your heart.
- Choose foods and nutrients from list **A** and help burn fat.
- Choose foods and nutrients from list **R** and lower and stabilize blood sugar.
- Choose foods and nutrients from list **T** and lower your cholesterol.

It's as easy as following your heart.

HEAL YOUR BLOOD PRESSURE

Research indicates that the following
nutrients reduce blood pressure

Fruits & Berries
- Bananas
- Blueberries
- Prunes
- Raisins
- Raspberries
- Strawberries
- Watermelon

Beans
- Black
- Kidney
- Lima
- Navy
- Pinto
- Soy
- White

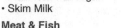

Nuts, Seeds & Oils
- Almonds
- Olive Oil
- Unsalted Sunflower Seeds

Dairy
- Low-fat Cottage Cheese
- Plain Non-Fat Yogurt
- Skim Milk

**Whole Grain &
High Fiber Cereals**
- Bran Flakes
- Oatmeal
- Sherdded Wheat

Meat & Fish
- Halibut

Spices, Herbs & Teas
- Spices
  Cardamom
  Cinnamon
  Garlic
- Herbs
  Hawthorn
  Oregano
- Tea
  Hibiscus

Vegetables
- Baked Potatoes
  (Purple)
- Beets
- Beet Juice
- Cabbage
- Carrots
- Lettuce
- Onions
- Spinach

Other
Dark Chocolate
(70% Cocoa Powder)

Avoid items that increase your blood pressure. Examples include: salt,
alcohol, high sodium processed foods such as pretzels, chips, canned soup,
dried soup mixes, bouillon, sausage, bacon, ham, fatty meats, peanuts,
popcorn, pickled goods, deli meats, prepared microwave meals, breads,
fast food, fried food, butter, and margarine.

ENERGIZE YOUR HEART

Research indicates that the following nutrients
energize your heart

Fruits & Berries
- Apples
- Bananas
- Mandarin
- Oranges

Nuts, Seeds & Oils
- Peanuts
- Peanut Butter
- Walnuts

**Whole Grain &
High Fiber Cereals**
- Oat Bran
- Oat Groats
- Oatmeal
- Quinoa

Vegetables
- Asparagus
- Broccoli
- Spinach

Beans
- Black
- Cannellini
- Garbanzo
- Green
- Haricot
- Kidney
- Lentils
- Lima (Butter)
- Mung
- Pinto
- Soy
- String

Dairy
- Eggs
- Low-Fat Cheese
  (Cheddar)
- Low-Fat Milk
- Low-Fat Yogurt

Meat & Fish
- Salmon

Spices, Herbs & Teas
Ginseng
- American Ginseng
  (Panax Quinquefolius)
- Asian Ginseng
  (Panax Ginseng)
- Eleuthero or
  Siberian Ginseng
  (Eleutherococcus
  Senticosus)
Herbs
- Schisandra
  (Shisandra Chinensis)
- Rhodiola
  (Rhodiola Rosea)

Supplements
- D-ribose
- Co-enzyme Q10
  (CoQ10)

Avoid items that slow metabolism. Examples include: white bread, pasta,
white rice, white flower, de-germed cornmeal sugar, fried food, fast food, cakes,
candy, cookies, canned fruit, soft drinks, beef, pork, butter, cheese, cream, milk,
canned foods, lunch meat, sausage, seasoned salt, meat tenderizers, ketchup,
mustard, salad dressing, salted peanuts, and commercially prepared meals.

A   ACT ON FAT

Research indicates that the following nutrients burn fat

Fruits & Berries

- Apples
- Avocados
- Bananas
- Blueberries
- Cantaloupe
- Garcinia Cambogia
- Grapefruit
- Grapes
- Oranges
- Peaches
- Pears
- Pineapple
- Strawberries

Nuts, Seeds & Oils
Nuts & Seeds
- Almonds
- Chia
- Flaxseeds
- Walnuts

Oils
- Canola
- Flaxseed
- Olive
- Soy

Vegetables
- Arugala
- Asparagus
- Bell Peppers
  (Green & Red)
- Broccoli
- Cabbage
- Cucumbers
- Endive
- Fennel
- Kale
- Mushrooms
- Onions
- Organic Leafy Greens
- Purslane
- Spinach
- Sweet Potatoes
- Tomatoes
- Yams
- Zucchini

Beans
- Black
- Cannellini
- Chickpeas
- Garbanzo
- Green
- Haricot
- Legumes
- Lentils

Dairy
- Eggs
- Fat-free or Low-fat Milk
- Fat-free or Low-fat Yogurt

Meat & Fish
Fish

- Mackerel
- Salmon
- Tilapia,
- Trout
- Tuna,

Meat
- Beef
- Bison/buffalo
- Chicken Breast
- Turkey Breast

Spices, Herbs & Teas
Spices
- Cayenne
- Chili Pepper
  (Red or Green)
- Curry
- Habanero
- Jalapeno
- Spicy Peppers

Teas
- Green
- Oolong

Coffee
- Green coffee bean

Supplements
- Casein Protein
- Whey Protein

Avoid nutrients that have high glycemic index (gi) and reduce fat burning.
Examples include: white bread, white rice, crackers, chips, bagels, cereal,
soft drinks, white potatoes, beer, cake, and corn syrup.

REDUCE YOUR BLOOD SUGAR

Research indicates that the following nutrients
stabilize your blood sugar

Fruits & Berries
- Avocados
- Bitter Melon
- Cherries
- Grapefruit
- Okra
- Lemons

Nuts, Seeds & Oils
Nuts & Seeds
- Almonds
- Brazil Nuts
- Cashews
- Macadamia Nuts
- Pecans
- Walnuts
- Flaxseeds

**Whole Grains &
High Fiber Cereals**
- Barley
- Oatmeal

Spices, Herbs & Teas
- Cinnamon
- Yarrow

Supplements
Brewers Yeast

Vegetables
- Broccoli
- Cabbage
- Garlic
- Leafy Greens
- Leeks
- Mitake Mushrooms
- Nopal
- Onions
- Peas
- Romaine Lettuce
- Spinach
- Sweet Potatoes
- White Potatoes
- Yams

Beans
- Black
- Cannellini
- Garbanzo
- Green
- Haricot
- Kidney
- Lentils
- Lima or Butter
- Mung
- Pinto
- Soy
- String

Avoid items with processed sugars and carbohydrates. Examples include
candy, high fructose corn syrup, sugar, brown sugar, glucose, dextrose, fructose,
fruit juice concentrates, molasses, syrup, soda, energy drinks, baked goods, cereals,
ice cream, jams, jellies, pasta, pizza, bread, and chips.

TACKLE TRIGLYCERIDES

Research indicates that the following nutrients
lower your cholesterol

Fruits & Berries
• Apples
• Citrus fruits
• Grapes
• Okra
• Pears
• Prunes
• Strawberries

Nuts, Seeds & Oils
Nuts & Seeds
• Almonds
• Pecans
• Walnuts
• Celery seeds
• Flaxseeds
• Psyllium seeds
Oils
• Canola
• Olive
• Safflower
• Sunflower

**Whole Grains &
High Fiber Cereals**
• Barley
• Oatmeal
• Oat Brans
• Prunes

Vegetables
• Eggplant,
• Jerusalem Artichoke
  (Sunchoke)

Beans
• Black Soybeans
• Kidney
• Lentils

Dairy
• Goat's Milk
• Greek Yogurt

Meat & Fish
• Albacore Tuna
• Halibut Mackerel
• Herring
• Lake Trout
• Salmon
• Sardines

Spices, Herbs & Teas
• Turmeric

Supplements
• Plant Sterols or Stanols

Other
• Soy
• Tempeh

Avoid items that increase your cholesterol such as "trans" fats. Examples
include: margarine, shortening, butter, cake mixes, frosting, other mixes (e.g.
Bisquick), dry soups, fast food, fried foods, frozen pies, frozen pie crust, frozen
pot pies, frozen waffles, frozen pizzas, frozen breaded fish sticks, ice cream,
non-dairy creamers, microwave popcorn, ground beef, cookies, biscuits, sweet
rolls, breakfast sandwiches, frozen or creamy beverages, meat sticks, crackers,
Asian crunchy noodles, canned chili, and packaged pudding.

Recipes

Jesse Schenker Recipes

30-year-old Jesse Schenker has amassed an impressive culinary history on his way to becoming Executive Chef and Owner of Recette, the urban, contemporary restaurant which he opened with his wife Lindsay, in New York's Greenwich Village in January of 2010. Just months after opening, Recette received two-star reviews from both the *New York Times* and *New York* Magazine.

Jesse has garnered numerous distinctions, including Best New Chef *New York* Magazine, Best New Restaurant the *New York Times*, "America's Best Young Chefs" in *Details* magazine, and Zagat's "30 Hottest Chefs Under 30" list. Recette was named "One of NYC's ten most exciting restaurants" by *Manhattan Magazine*. Additional accomplishments include *Forbes*'s "30 Under 30" in the food and wine industry in December 2011, as well as Schenker's recent victorious battle on the Food Network's *Iron Chef America*.

Jesse was a James Beard Semifinalist Nominee for Rising Star Chef and Best New Restaurant in 2011.

Read more about Jesse at www.jesseschenker.com.

Here are two delicious recipes created by Jesse that include ingredients from the 5 for 1 diet.

Barley Risotto with Baked Salmon

    H—Olive Oil
    E—Salmon
    A—Walnut
    R—Lemon
    T—Greek Yogurt

RISOTTO

    1 c barley
    ½ c Greek yogurt
    1 tbsp olive oil
    2 cups water
    1 tbsp salt
    Pinch pepper
    1 pc lemon
    1 sprig Italian Parsley
    ¼ toasted walnut

In medium sauce pan over medium heat, pour 1 tbsp olive oil then add the dry barley, cook the barley for about 2 minutes to get a little nutty flavor in grain. Add water a little bit at a time. Try the barley like you cook real risotto rice. Repeat process until the barley is cooked.. Lastly fold in the Greek yogurt, add a little splash of lemon juice, black pepper and adjust the seasoning to taste and chopped parsley.

Optional:
    Add toasted walnuts.

BAKED SALMON

Square foil, put 1/2 pound salmon, seasoned with salt and 3 slices lemons on top. Sealed the foil and baked it for 15 minutes

To Finish

Put the risotto barley on the bottom of the plate and baked salmon on top.

Chicken "Taco" Salad

H—Black Beans, Chili Powder
E—Jalapeno
A—Cucumber, Chicken
R—Onion
T—Greek Yogurt, Tomato

INGREDIENTS

2 chicken breasts (skinless)
¼ cup dry black beans
1 whole avocado
1 hot house cucumber
1 tbsp red onion
1 pc jalapeno
1 pc Roma tomato
1 bunch cilantro
½ c low fat Greek yogurt
2 pcs lime
1 tbsp salt
½ tsp black pepper
1 head iceburg lettuce (any green preference)
1 tsp chili powder

15 minutes prior to baking the chicken breast, marinate the breast with salt, pepper, and chili powder with lime juice. After 15 minutes bake the chicken breast in sheet tray and make sure to spread about 1 tbsp of olive oil on the tray to prevent it from sticking. Bake the chicken in the oven over 350 F for about 20 minutes, check to make sure it cooked all the way and let it rest.

In a medium saucepot with water boil the black beans with salt. Because the black beans take a while to cook it's advisable to cook the beans the night before or ahead of time before serving the salad. It makes it easier to just toss everything without the hassle of waiting for the beans to cook.

Cut the cucumber, tomatoes and avocado to medium dice (*Make sure to squeeze a little bit of lemon juice on top of the avocado to prevent it from oxidizing), thinly slice the jalapeno and red onion. Set all the vegetables aside. In a separate bowl, break the iceberg lettuce into a big piece. (Don't break it into small pieces since it will serve as the base of the salad.)

DRESSING

Finely chop the cilantro, put the chopped cilantro into a bowl then add the yogurt, salt and lime juice. Whisk it together. Adjust seasoning by adding more salt or lime juice.

To Finish

Slice chicken breast and set it aside. In a big bowl mix all the vegetables, black beans and the cilantro dressing. Adjust the seasoning to your liking.

On the bottom of the plate, place the iceburg lettuce, put the dressed vegetable and chicken breast on top.

Tofu Chicken Sandwich with Cucumber Kimchi, Lettuce Salad

H—Lettuce, Tofu

E—Egg

A—Cucumber

R—Garlic

T—Olive Oil

TOFU CHICKEN SANDWICH

Firm Tofu-1pack, from an Asian market if possible

Chicken breast-1ea, butterfly

Flour-½ cup

Egg-2ea

MARINATING INGREDIENTS

Onion-½ ea, medium, white, sliced

Garlic-2 cloves, thinly sliced

Olive oil-1cup

Black peppercorn-crushed

Lime juice-1ea

Salt-2 teaspoon

CUCUMBER KIMCHI

Kirby-5ea, cut in half lengthwise and deseeded

Garlic-3 cloves, minced

Rice wine vinegar-½cup

Korean chili powder (for kimchi)-⅔ cup

Sugar-½ cup

Salt-½ cup

Lettuce-Any type of leafy greens, cut into bite size

KIMCHI NON-FAT YOGURT SPREAD

Cucumber kimchi-1 cup

Non-fat yogurt-1 cup

Method

1. Take the tofu out of the package. Apply light pressure on to the top of tofu to remove any excess water, taking the extra moisture out.

2. Butterfly chicken breast and marinate with onion, garlic, olive oil, crushed black peppercorn, fresh lime juice and salt for about an hour.

3. Cut the Kirby cucumbers in half lengthwise, and deseed them. Slice them into even thickness (1/4inch) and salt them for about 20 minutes.

4. Once the excess moisture is removed from the tofu, cut them into 2-inch squares. Season the tofu with salt and lightly dust them all the way around with AP flour.

5. Grill the marinated chicken breast. Cut them into 2 inch squares.

6. Place the chicken breast between 2 pieces of tofu (just like making sandwich), and dip it in egg wash. Make sure the egg coats the entire sandwich.

7. Using a nonstick pan, sauté the sandwich in olive oil all the way around in a gentle heat. Once the egg sealed the entire sandwich, take it out of the pan.

8. Squeeze the moisture out of the cucumbers, and toss with remaining ingredients. Let it sit for about 30 minutes.

9. For kimchi non-fat yogurt spread, puree the ingredients together in a blender with pinch of salt.

Assemble

Cut the tofu chicken sandwich in half. Smear spoonful of kimchi non-fat yogurt on a plate. Place the sandwich on top of spread, cut side up. Toss the cucumber kimchi with lettuce and serve on side.

Grace O Recipes

Grace O is a friend, colleague and author of *Foodtrients: Age-Defying Recipes for a Sustainable Life*, and has been cooking and baking professionally and recreationally all of her adult life. As a child in Southeast Asia, she learned the culinary arts by her mother's side in her family's cooking school. She became so well versed in hospitality and the culinary arts, she eventually took over the cooking school and opened three restaurants. She is widely credited with popularizing shrimp on sugar-cane skewers and being one of the first chefs to make tapas a global trend. She has cooked for ruling families and royalty.

Grace O's move to America precipitated a career in healthcare, inspired by her father, who was a physician. Twenty years and much hard work later, she operates skilled nursing facilities in California.

Grace O's blog, *Aging Gracefully*, appears on FoodTrients.com. She is also a regular contributor to ScrubsMag.com, the award-winning lifestyle nursing magazine and website, and writes a regular column for the Asian Journal.

Here are two delicious recipes created by Grace that include ingredients from the *5 for 1 Diet*.

Baked Tilapia with Turmeric

H—olive oil
E—eggs
A—tilapia
R—Lemon
T—Turmeric

Turmeric juice makes this dish much more healthful. The Omega-3s in turmeric is known the world over for its amazing anti-inflammatory and anti-cancer benefits.

INGREDIENTS (SERVES 4)

⅓ cup fresh turmeric juice (see recipe below)
2 tbs mirin (seasoned rice wine)
Sea salt and ground pepper to taste
2 lbs. of tilapia fillets
3-4 beaten medium eggs
⅔ cup all-purpose flour
2-3 Tbs. olive oil

To make the marinade, combine the turmeric juice, mirin, salt, and pepper in a small bowl. Marinate the fillets in a covered dish in the refrigerator for 1 hour. Drain fillets from marinade and set aside. Add the reserved marinade to the eggs. Stir to combine. Dredge the fillets in the flour, and then dip in the egg mixture. Heat the olive oil in a large frying pan over medium-high heat. Add fillets and cook until golden brown, about 2-3 minutes on each side.

TURMERIC JUICE

¼ lb. turmeric root, peeled
½ cup water

Slice the turmeric root until it measures about 1 cup. Place the turmeric slices in a food processor or a blender. Add a bit of the water and blend at low speed. Gradually increase the speed, slowly adding water until all of the water is used up and mixture is smooth. Strain the juice using a fine-mesh strainer, cheesecloth, or coffee filter. Use lemon juice or a ¼ lemon wedge.

Spinach and Grapefruit Salad

H—garlic
E—spinach
A—chili powder
R—grapefruit
T—olive oil

Spinach contains iron as well as age-defying antioxidants. Grapefruit is chock-full of vitamin C and potassium. You can use pink or white grapefruit in this salad, though pink grapefruit has the added benefit of lycopene. If you use whole segments of the grapefruit, you'll also add fiber.

INGREDIENTS (SERVES 2)

1 bunch or 1 bag spinach leaves
1 whole grapefruit, segmented
¼ cup candied walnuts
¼ cup dried apricots

HONEY LIME DRESSING (SEE RECIPE BELOW)

Wash and stem the spinach leaves and place in bowl. Add the grapefruit, walnuts, and apricots. Toss with honey lime dressing to taste.

HONEY-LIME DRESSING

This is a very versatile dressing that you can toss with my Spinach and Grapefruit Salad. The lime juice provides vitamin C, while compounds in the chili powder help to neutralize free radicals in your cells. If you want a spicier dressing, add cayenne pepper or red pepper flakes. Both contain capsaicin, which stimulates circulation. To use this dressing with fruit salad, simply omit the allicin-rich garlic—it will still be nutritious!

INGREDIENTS (YIELDS ¼ CUP)

1 ½ Tbs. lime juice (about 1 lime)
1 ½ Tbs. honey

1 Tbs. extra-virgin olive oil
1 minced garlic clove
½ tsp. chili powder
Sea salt to taste

   Combine all the ingredients in a container with a tight-fitting lid and shake until well blended.

Turkey Chili

INGREDIENTS:

   1 lb. ground lean turkey (A)

   1 onion (finely chopped) (H, A, R)

   1 bell pepper (finely chopped) (A)

   2 Portobello mushroom caps (finely chopped) (A)

   3 cloves garlic (finely chopped) (H, R)

   1 15 oz. can corn

   1 15 oz. can black beans (H, E, A, R)

   1 15 oz. can tomato sauce

   1 28 oz. can diced tomatoes (A)

   Avocado (A, R)

   Greek Yogurt (T)

   2-tablespoon olive oil (H, A, T)

   1 tsp. cumin

   2 tsp. chili powder (A)

   2 tsp. red pepper flakes (A)

Put 2-tbsp olive oil in a pot. Sauté finely chopped onion, bell pepper, portabella mushrooms, and garlic until just beginning to brown. Add a pinch of salt and pepper. Remove vegetables from pot. Add 1 lb. ground lean turkey to pot. Break apart and season with 1 tsp. cumin, 2 tsp. chili powder and 2 tsp. red pepper flakes. Add a little salt and pepper. Once turkey is nearly cooked add corn, black beans, tomato sauce, diced tomatoes, and Sautéed veggies. Stir to combine. Reduce heat to medium low. Simmer for approximately 20 min. Salt and pepper to taste. Serve with Greek yogurt and Avocado.

JOHN KENNEDY RECIPES

Grilled Salmon & Zucchini with Red Pepper Sauce

H—⅓ cup sliced almonds, toasted

E—1 ¼ pounds wild-caught salmon fillet, skinned and cut crosswise into 4 portions

A—2 medium zucchini, or summer squash (or 1 of each), halved lengthwise

¼ cup chopped jarred roasted red peppers

¼ cup halved grape tomatoes, or cherry tomatoes

R—1 small clove garlic

T—1-tbsp extra-virgin olive oil

1 tbsp chopped fresh parsley, for garnish

1 tbsp sherry vinegar, or red-wine vinegar

1 tsp paprika, preferably smoked

¾ tsp salt, divided

½ tsp freshly ground pepper, divided

DIRECTIONS

Preheat grill to medium. Process almonds, peppers, tomatoes, garlic, oil, vinegar, paprika ¼ tsp salt and ¼ tsp pepper in a food processor or blender until smooth; set aside. Coat salmon and zucchini (and/or) summer squash on both sides with cooking spray, then sprinkle with the remaining ½ tsp salt and ¼ tsp pepper. Grill, turning once, until the salmon is just cooked through and the squash is soft and browned, about 3 minutes per side. Transfer the squash to a clean cutting board. When cool enough to handle, slice into ½ -inch pieces. Toss in a bowl with half of the reserved sauce. Divide the squash among 4 plates along with a piece of salmon topped with some of the remaining sauce. Garnish with parsley, if desired.

Tips:

To toast chopped or sliced nuts, stir constantly in a small dry skillet over medium-low heat until fragrant and lightly browned, 2 to 4 minutes.

To skin a salmon fillet, place on a clean cutting board, skin side down. Starting at the tail end, slip the blade of a long, sharp knife between the fish flesh and the skin, holding the skin down firmly with your other hand. Gently push the blade along at a 30-degree angle, separating the fillet from the skin without cutting through either.

PART III

A Heart Healthy Future

CHAPTER 10

Kids: Learn 5 Early and Prevent 5 Later

Take a survey. You'll certainly find that most people only think of older adults as being affected by heart disease. And heart disease is the leading cause of death among adults age 50 and over. Yet, the multiple risk factors that contribute to cardiovascular illness, including obesity, lack of physical activity, diabetes, and high cholesterol levels, are showing up earlier in life. Today, almost five million children age 12 to 17 smoke; almost 50 percent of kids don't exercise regularly; and an estimated 33 percent of U.S. children are overweight or obese.[1,2] Many readers of this book will be parents, and every reader once was once a child. Thus, the advice and guidance in this chapter will interest every one of us. While some childhood heart problems can't be prevented, heart-healthy lifestyle choices and habits such as proper nutrition, regular exercise, and maintaining a healthy weight should start early, as this is the clearest path to prevent cardiovascular problems in adulthood. As a cautionary tale, I share a poignant and these days all-too-familiar story of a critically ill patient whose parents ignored the warnings signs and even their own intuitive sense that their daughter's cardiovascular health was at risk. Drawing on my own experience as a parent and founder of the *Big Mind, Brave Heart, Bright Future Campaign*—a program designed to help kids cope with stress and prevent future heart disease—I emphasize the significance of the five steps, and offer his strategies and advice of talking to children about the importance of living a heart healthy lifestyle. Anyone who has children and anyone who has been a child will find a wealth of valuable guidance in this chapter.

GARTH AND MARY: ALL IN THE GENES?

Few things filled Mary with more pride than her ten-year-old son, Garth. At the drop of a hat she would pull out the photo album she'd been carrying in her purse since the day she first brought him home from the hospital. Mary never grew tired of regaling her co-workers with stories of her only child's straight-A report cards, his Chess Club exploits, or the Saturday afternoons he'd spend volunteering at a local animal shelter.

After her husband's untimely death, Mary doted heavily on Garth, doing her best to fill in the gaps. Of course, no one can be in two places at once, and Mary struggled to balance her obligations at work with the responsibility of caring for a ten-year-old boy. Most nights, she'd leave work promptly at 5 and drive over to Garth's school, where he'd pass the time doing homework, playing with friends, or participating in some sort of enrichment program. At home, Mary never had to remind Garth to do his homework. Typically, he finished it at school anyway. Since he didn't have anything he needed to do after returning home—other than helping his mother set the table or take out the trash—he'd often pass the time playing video games. Mary didn't love her son's nonstop gaming but she already felt badly about having to put him in an afterschool program. And since he was such a good kid, she didn't see any need to crack the whip. They were just video games after all.

While Mary didn't seem that concerned with Garth's video game obsession, she did notice that he'd started to put on weight in recent months. And not just a pound or two, but what she described to a friend as a "significant" amount of weight. "I'm concerned about Garth. He's really packing on the pounds," she said.

Naturally, Mary wondered if there was a correlation between the amount of time Garth was spending playing video games and his sudden, rapid weight gain. She was familiar with all the reports, including a study Garth's pediatrician had shared about the link between excessive video game playing and increased calorie consumption. She didn't think it was good idea to ban video games altogether, knowing that might alienate Garth and take away an important emotional outlet. Plus, he was keeping up his good grades, so clearly his fondness for gaming wasn't getting in the way of his schoolwork. She even thought of investing in Wii Fit, since it would allow her to interact more with her sedentary son and get them both more involved in a healthy physical activity. "If he's moving while he's gaming then he won't have time to snack," she reasoned.

One thing Mary and Garth enjoyed doing together was looking through family photo albums. Family photos made Mary feel better, at least for a few moments, and helped her make sense of her husband's sudden passing a year earlier. Garth also benefited since he was nine when his father died, old enough to have a sense of who he was. On the first anniversary of her husband's death, Mary happened to be looking through her wedding album when a startling revelation came to mind. In every sense of the word, Garth was the spitting image of her late husband, right down to his mop of curly brown hair and slightly dimpled chin. "A real mini-me," she thought. Not only did they physically resemble each other, but Garth's father also was obese, sedentary, and an avid video gamer. In fact, they'd spend hours playing games together. Angry Birds Rio was their personal favorite.

The uncanny resemblance caused Mary to wonder if her son's weight problem was all in his "genes." She scheduled an appointment with the pediatrician. During the visit, Mary received some startling news. "Mary, there's no way to couch this, so I'm just going to say it. Garth has gained more than 100 pounds since his last visit less than a year ago. His BMI is over 30. In other words, he's medically obese. Moreover, he shared that he'd been drinking a lot and urinating frequently, and he's tired and hungry all the time." Unbeknownst to Mary, Garth also had developed a small velvety rash on his neck, a telltale sign of diabetes. "I won't know for sure until we get his blood work back but all the signs point to diabetes," he added.

The news hit Mary like a ton of bricks. She felt personally responsible for her son's startling weight gain and deteriorating health. "I can't believe I let his happen," a distraught Mary told the pediatrician. Quickly, her anguish turned to worry. She remembered reading about a 218-pound 8-year-old Ohio boy who was removed from his home and placed in foster care because he was considered too fat. Would the same thing happen to her? Would the pediatrician contact Child Protective Services and have her son removed from the only home he'd ever known?

"Take it easy Mary. No one is taking away your son," the pediatrician assured Mary. "But I wouldn't be fulfilling my obligation to Garth and to you if I didn't say up front that he's severely obese and his weight has put him at risk for developing a host of illnesses, including childhood diabetes, high blood pressure, and even heart disease," he added.

The issue of kids and weight and who's responsible is a thorny subject. It may seem odd to some, hypocritical even, that our government would consider removing overweight kids from their homes while simultaneously saying that it's fine to advertise unhealthy, non-nutritious food and even put toys in fast food meals as an enticement to buy and consume more and more. As a cardiologist, I'm not here to argue that weight isn't a problem for millions of kids. It is a problem. Indeed, it's been estimated that 33 percent of children under the age of 17 are obese and my personal feeling is that the number is much higher.[3] But when does weight become an imminent danger to a child? Removing Garth from his home wouldn't help. His mother was one of the nicest, most well-intentioned parents I've ever run across. Clearly, Garth would suffer far more by being removed from his mother's care than remaining in a home at an unhealthy weight. As an interesting aside, there are multiple negative mental and physical health consequences from being in foster care, including a 35 percent increase in BMI.[4]

Still, the status quo couldn't continue. As I told Mary when she came in with Garth for a consult, "Even though your son is young, he is at risk and on a dangerous path that will greatly impact his future. I know you're juggling a lot of balls but we need to do something about his weight." If Garth continued on this path, he almost certainly faced a lifetime of serious and even life-threatening health concerns, as his pediatrician had alluded to earlier. I stressed the importance of intervening now, while Garth was still young since it's known that child obesity is rooted in poor eating habits that began as early as age twelve to twenty-four months. Poor habits such as frequent high-calorie in-between-meal snacks profoundly affect a child's later eating habits and his or her weight. As *New York Times'* bestselling author Michael Pollan observed in his critically acclaimed book, *Cooked: A Natural History of Transformation*, Americans spend seventy-eight minutes a day in secondary eating and drinking, which is more time than they spend on meals or primary eating.[5,6]

Mary was a fighter. She had survived a lot in her thirty-eight years, including the deaths of her husband and older sister. She wasn't about to take this news lying down. Once the reality of Garth's condition had sunk in, she sprang into action. Mary cut back on the long hours at work. As a marketing manager for a pharmaceutical company, she could make her own schedule. As long as the work got done, or she wasn't meeting with a client, she could work from home. She started preparing Garth's lunch, instead of giving him money to buy it at school. She started limiting his video game time to ½ hour a day and instituted a "no snack rule" while he was playing. Mary also became active in the PTA, and lobbied local politicians about the importance of having healthy food options available for school kids.

As she got more and more involved in her passion project, it struck her just how physically inactive a majority of kids were at Garth's school. Looking into the matter further, she discovered that physical education classes had been cut dramatically in the face of anemic local tax collections and dropping property values and that students were being granted little or no time in the gym. In fact, the local school district hadn't even filed a physical education plan with the state in five years.

Mary was so shocked by the cuts in physical education classes that she organized a grass-roots effort designed to mount political pressure to reverse the cuts. With the support of the PTA, Mary helped organize several school health initiatives, including daily fifteen-minute "exercise breaks" in classrooms and before-and-after-school for all elementary school students. A year after the program started, a fitness assessment was given to the town's kindergarten through fifth-grade students, showing a 7 percent drop in the number of obese kids, the biggest decline reported by any town or city in the state.

Mary's new mission so inspired her that she penned a heartfelt letter to President Obama about her personal experience with childhood obesity. Mary's letter was brought to the attention of First Lady Michelle Obama, who was so impressed that she made her an official spokesperson and public advocate for her "Let's Move" campaign aimed at curbing childhood obesity. Back home, Mary's newfound celebrity prompted several local merchants to jump on the bandwagon and donate money to fund the construction of a brand new school gymnasium and create an afterschool sports program. Several local restaurants also got involved, agreeing to donate healthy food for school lunches. An ad hoc group of nutritionists and doctors volunteered their time to teach kids about the importance of healthy food choices and regular physical activity.

A SAD LANDSCAPE

Mary and Garth's story, as extreme as Garth's weight gain and subsequent health problems were, shines a light on a critical issue vexing our society: childhood obesity.

As a preventive and interventional cardiologist, it's now a sad reality of my job that I see obese children almost daily in my office. When I began my medical career, two decades ago, I could never have envisioned such a scenario. What's happened in the intervening twenty years? Why are younger and younger children showing up in my office?

Whenever I give a talk about kids and heart disease I always get more than my fair share of blank stares and incredulous looks. "These are kids, Dr. Kennedy. Why are you talking to them about heart disease?" It never crosses the minds of most parents that their happy, active seven-year-old could have the heart of a sixty-year-old man. Of course, most "active" seven-year-olds do not have this problem. And therein lies the dilemma. Increasingly, we're seeing more and more kids acquire unhealthy habits that increase their risk for cardiovascular disease later in life. Cardiovascular disease starts early and has a long asymptomatic lag time, putting the vast numbers of children in this country who are overweight or obese at risk.

Of greatest concern to me is the duration of obesity, particularly when the problem begins in childhood, and how it affects heart disease risk. Basically, the longer you're fat, the greater risk of CAD. A study of 3,200 young adults, ages 18–30 concluded that exclusive of

BMI and waist circumference, for every year of obesity the risk of developing silent heart disease increases by 2–4 percent.[7]

THE SKINNY ON HEART DISEASE IN CHILDREN

Congenital

Basically, we see two types of heart disease in children: Congenital and acquired. Congenital heart defects are present at birth and are typically present with an abnormally structured heart and/or large vessels. Examples might include a heart with incomplete or missing parts, a heart that hasn't been assembled correctly, a heart with holes between chamber partitions, or a heart with narrow or leaky valves or narrow vessels. There are many types of congenital heart defects, ranging from those that pose relatively small threats to the health of the child such as atrial septal defect to those that require immediate surgery like ventricular septal defect.

Pioneering technology like the Level II ultrasound and a fetal echocardiogram have enabled us to detect some in-utero CHDs. After birth, congenital heart disease is often first detected when the doctor hears an abnormal heart sound or murmur when listening to the heart. Depending on the type of murmur, he or she may order further testing such as Echocardiogram, Cardiac catheterization, Chest X-Ray, Electrocardiogram (ECG/EKG), Magnetic Resonance Imaging (MRI) or other diagnostic testing.

The warning signs of congenital heart disease in infants and children may include a heart murmur or abnormal heart sound, cyanosis—a bluish tint to the skin, fingernails and/or lips—fast breathing, poor eating habits, underweight, an inability to exercise and excessive sweating.

Acquired

Acquired heart disease is the second type of heart problem that occurs in children. This problem appears after birth. It takes two

DEAD RINGER

Early in my career, I had two patients: 28-year-old identical twins brothers, with a long family history of premature coronary artery disease. The twins' parents and all of their paternal and maternal uncles died of the disease by age thirty. One brother, Armando, was your typical type-A overachiever. An incredibly successful stockbroker but also a compulsive workaholic, Armando never gave much thought to fourteen-hour days, all while chained to desk, chain smoking cigarettes, and wolfing down cheeseburgers and French fries for lunch. Armando's only exercise consisted of a short stroll from the elevator to his plush office suite. That plush suite—the scene of so much heart unhealthy behavior—was his undoing, as Armando's personal assistant arrived early one morning to find her boss dead, his face, in a moment of poetic justice, planted squarely in a large black ashtray that sat on top of his large pristine oak desk. Ironically, Armando had died while talking to his brother Raphael about making major lifestyle changes.

Armando's death hit Raphael hard. As he sat in my office a month after the funeral, Raphael talked about his brother's unhealthy lifestyle. Like Armando, Raphael was a successful stockbroker. Unlike Armando, Raphael was a gym rat, followed a mostly vegetarian diet, and began each day meditating before commuting by ferry to his office in downtown San Francisco. He was keenly aware of his long family history of CAD, and following his brother's death, thought it would be wise to get himself checked out. It was a good call. A stress test revealed a blocked coronary artery. Since Raphael was asymptomatic, I was able to treat him with Aspirin and a cholesterol-lowering medication. Today, Raphael continues his heart healthy lifestyle and stops by for regular checkups. Ten years after his brother's death and Raphael is still symptom free, suggesting a healthy lifestyle decreased the progression of his disease and may have reversed it altogether.

forms. Usually it is the result of damage done to the heart by a disease, virus, or bacteria. Rheumatic fever, an inflammatory disorder of the body's connective tissue that's triggered by a Group A strep throat infection or scarlet fever, is the most common acquired heart problem seen in children. It can cause temporary but painful arthritis, small, painless nodules under the skin, fatigue, swollen joints and in the worst case scenario, shortness of breath and chest pain—and a possible indication of heart problems.

In some children with acquired heart disease, a cause cannot be found—known as a "diagnosis of exclusion." This is the case with idiopathic dilated cardiomyopathy, a condition in which the heart becomes weakened and enlarged and cannot pump blood efficiently. Kawasaki disease is another example of acquired heart disease that causes blockages in the coronary arteries and is probably autoimmune mediated. Though genetics may play a role, if there is no other relative with congenital heart disease, the risk is only slightly greater.

There is a significant difference between heart disease—congenital or acquired—that affects children and the type of heart disease that affects adults. Adults have coronary artery disease that may cause heart attacks. Heart disease that affects children is different from coronary artery disease and rarely causes heart attacks.

The Other "Acquired" Heart Disease

By now, we all know the factors that combine to give us a healthy heart. Controlling high blood pressure, regular physical activity, eating a diet consisting of heart healthy foods, maintaining an ideal weight, and controlling cholesterol and blood sugar. But it's been suggested that only half of U.S. kids meet just four or fewer of these heart health criteria.

The Centers for Disease Control and Prevention (CDC) found that one in five children had abnormal cholesterol levels, leading to a recommendation by the American Academy of Pediatrics that all children nine to eleven years old be screened for high cholesterol levels.[8] The CDC also reports that a third of American children are currently overweight or obese, putting them at an increased risk for cardiovascular disease.

It's rare for children to show signs of atherosclerosis, yet more and more children are showing up in doctors' offices—mine included—with vascular changes similar to those seen in adults. It shouldn't come as much of a surprise since elevated cholesterol, pre-diabetes, high blood pressure, physical inactivity, and exposure to cigarette smoke are now a part of daily life for far too many children. High triglyceride-to-HDL ratio has been linked to arterial stiffness in adults, and now that same lethal combination has touched the lives of kids.

FALLING ON DEAF EARS

If any group would benefit the most from a prevention model, you'd think it would be kids. What better time to intervene than childhood before symptoms even start? Lifestyle change, including diet, exercise, and stress reduction, is the go-to remedy, which makes sense, although it poses major challenges. How, as an example, can we convince kids to reduce their consumption of sugary beverages, which contribute greatly to elevated blood sugar and triglyceride levels and obesity, when Spider-Man, Minnie Mouse and Lightning McQueen are telling them it's perfectly OK to suck down a 6 oz. juice box that has almost half the RDA of sugar? Who's the average 9-year-old going to listen to? Even a single serving cup of a popular yogurt brand contains most of the total daily allowance of sugar recommended by the American Heart Association for Children.

In the battle against food companies for the hearts, minds, and stomachs of our nation's youth, well-intentioned parents, healthcare professionals, and educators are clearly outnumbered and outgunned. According to a 2012 report from the FTC, in 2009 food and beverage companies spent almost $1.8 billion marketing directly to children between the ages of two to seven.[9] Interactive game websites for kids, Internet advertising, sponsorships at sporting events and amusement parks, vending machines in school cafeterias and product placement in movies, video games and TV shows are just some of the ways food advertisers now reach kids. Fast-food restaurants, which already cough up $10 billion marketing directly to children, now place banner and pop up ads on mobile websites, smartphone applications, and text messaging ads. Even celebrities are getting into the act, with some of this country's best-known athletes and actors shilling everything from fast food restaurant chains to soft drinks. Celebrity endorsements in particular are a powerful and effective method for creating value, recognition, and credibility for a particular food or brand. But I don't need a published study to tell me that celebrity endorsement of a food encourages children to eat more. Pepsi didn't pay Beyoncé $50 million to endorse their products because they like the way she sings.

The food industry weaves its web, in part, by targeting your children via a strategy commonly known as "pester power," a form of "marketing that enlists young children as third parties to influence adult parents to purchase unhealthy food and beverages," according to an issue brief from The Public Health Advocacy Institute.[10] It seems to be doing the trick since the average toddler sees nearly three fast-food advertisements every day; kids ages six to eleven view three-and-a-half ads daily; and teenagers, nearly five, according to a study by Yale's Rudd Center for Obesity & Public Policy.[11]

B THE NUMBERS; ASSESSING YOUR CHILD'S RISK

Problems notwithstanding, heart disease still isn't a major cause of death and disability among children. And most of the risk factors that affect children—high blood pressure, high cholesterol, smoking, obesity and physical inactivity—can be controlled early in life. Particularly with children, prevention is the best way to avoid problems later on.

High Blood Pressure

First, some good news: High blood pressure affects fewer than 3 percent of U.S. children. Hypertension in children isn't a congenital disease, but there may be a genetic correlation. Most cases of hypertension in children are the result of other diseases, a phenomenon we refer to as secondary hypertension. Children rarely have primary hypertension. In most instances, high blood pressure in children can be treated with simple lifestyle modifications such as healthy weight loss, increased physical activity, limiting salt and sugar intake, and repeated admonitions about the dangers of smoking.

Cholesterol

Only a small percentage of children have high cholesterol, or plaque buildup—known as "fatty streaks"—that begins early and progresses slowly. Left untreated, plaque buildup leads to atherosclerosis. Most often when I see high cholesterol in kids, particularly if they don't have any other obvious risk factors, then I always suspect genes are in play, as they were with my patient Anna, whose experience with familial hypercholesterolemia opened Chapter 4. Still, high cholesterol is rare, affecting just 1 to 2 percent of children. I tell parents that unless their kids have all the known risk factors, then it's not necessary to have cholesterol screening until their late teens (AAP guidelines notwithstanding). Guidelines for controlling cholesterol in kids are no different from those of adults:

- Regular, vigorous exercise for at least thirty minutes (but preferably sixty minutes) four to five days a week
- A diet low in saturated fat, and high in simple carbohydrates
- Awareness about the dangers of cigarette smoking

- Finding a healthy, livable weight, which is directly tied to diet and exercise
- Only rarely are kids with cholesterol prescribed medication.

Smoking

The dangers of smoking should be obvious to everyone. But every day, nearly 4,000 kids under age eighteen light up for the first time. Most smokers—90 percent—start before they finish high school. It's been estimated for the children who would otherwise be at very low risk, smoking may account for 75 percent of heart disease cases.[12] Smoking increases both the risk of heart disease and peripheral vascular disease since nicotine narrows and hardens the blood vessels. Other chemicals in cigarettes may also damage the heart. High blood pressure, fatty plaque buildup and blood clots have all been linked to smoking (the chemicals in cigarettes increase fibrinogen levels, a blood clotting material).

Warning children about the dangers of cigarette smoking is a vexing problem for adults. I tell parents to appeal to their children's vanity. Discuss the "noticeable" effects of smoking like yellow teeth, bad breath, yellow skin, saggy skin, and smelly clothes. This is an approach I've found especially helpful with appearance obsessed teens. Most important, be a role model for your kids. If you smoke, quit immediately. Here's a number to consider: If smoking rates continue apace, 5 million teens will die of smoking related diseases.[13]

Obesity

Among children, obesity and overweight are the biggest risk factors for heart disease. It's believed that up to 33 percent of U.S. children are obese, explaining why we're seeing an increase in weight related diseases like type-2 diabetes among young people. Here's another frightening fact: Obese and overweight children are more likely to be obese and overweight adults. Obesity and overweight is especially dangerous in children since the fat cells we acquired in childhood become our lifelong companions. Weight loss decreases the size but not the number of fat cells. I advise parents who are concerned about their children's weight to use the same BMI calculator used for adults. To find your children's BMI percentile, follow the link listed in the resource section of the book.

Since obesity is becoming increasing prevalent among American children, and showing up in younger ages, I believe that along with BMI and waist circumference, we should consider obesity duration, since the longer a kid is fat the more likely he or she is to develop heart disease. If you're worried about your child's weight, the first thing you should do is visit your healthcare provider to make sure the weight gain isn't the result of an underlying medical problem such as hypothyroidism, edema stemming from a heart, kidney or liver problem, or Cushing's syndrome.

Below are some of favorite strategies for pointing kids in the direction of healthy weight control.

- Avoid the "food as a reward or motivation" trap (Johnny, I'll buy you ice cream if you do your homework). In the long run, that strategy always backfires. You don't want kids associating food with a reward, or goodie for a job well done.
- Pack your child's lunch instead of giving her money to buy it at school.
- No eating while watching television and seriously consider limiting the time they spend watching TV, or playing on the computer or iPad.
- Control their portion sizes.
- If possible, eat at least one meal a day as a family.
- Set aside time for regular physical activity, especially as a family.

Physical Activity

In an era of high technology, convincing kids that a vigorous soccer game is preferable to an hour of Angry Birds Rio is no easy feat. But we need to. Physically inactive kids are likely to become physically inactive adults. And they're setting the stage for a lifetime of heart disease risk factors including high cholesterol, diabetes, obesity and high blood pressure.

Regular exercise has so many benefits for kids that it's almost impossible to list them all here. But improvements in cardiovascular health, including lowered blood pressure, increase in HDL cholesterol, and reduction of stress are reasons enough to encourage our children to make regular vigorous exercise part of their H-E-A-R-T healthy regimen.

You could be in for a challenge, especially if your child has grown up on a steady diet of X-Box and Grand Theft Auto. But I encourage you to set serious limits on the time spent watching TV, playing video games, or surfing the Internet. I've actually found that most kids respond well to limit setting. It provides a structure, clear boundaries and a sense of safety. It's also a strategy for keeping them away from the onslaught of food advertising geared directly toward kids.

Look into organized exercise such as dance or gymnastics classes or a sports team. Schedule regular weekly family outings that involve a type of physical activity. I set aside time each week to hike the hills outside Los Angeles with my daughters. Remember to keep the activity playful and fun so they don't associate physical activity with a chore, and will be more inclined to continue exercising in the future.

Stress

We all have bad habits—annoying unconscious things we do without much thought but are probably infuriating to those around us. Whether the habit is harmless or harmful, one thing triggers nearly every habit I can think of: Stress.

Peer, parents, academics, athletics—there's an endless number of forces that apply performance pressure to our kids. To cope, some kids seek comfort in bad habits—overeating, smoking, and drinking to list a handful. Stress-induced bad habits can be a first step on the path to heart disease.

Stress chips away at children's self-control and resolve. For kids, that reality can manifest in many ways. Kids who find their willpower depleted by stress may adopt or return to bad habits. Think about it. When stressed, do you reach for a carrot, apple, slice of low-fat cheese, or the nearest jelly doughnut? They don't call doughnuts comfort foods for nothing.

With kids, it's important to start good habits early. If they snack at age seven, they're more likely to repeat that behavior at age twenty-six, even when stressed.

PARENTS: TAKING AN HONEST SELF-ASSESSMENT

The other day I was walking down the street with my daughters when we came upon a toy store. It must've just opened because I'm confident that after ten years of parenting I'd already visited every toy store within a hundred-mile radius of my house. Immediately, the store caught the interest of my children, particularly my youngest daughter, who was drawn to a rather large, not to mention expensive doll in the display window. Apparently, this doll was the hottest thing on the market and my daughter had to have it. "Daddy, please, please can we buy her?" I'll admit it; I'm not the toughest dad on the planet and my kids are terrific students and just good all-around people, so I have a hard time saying "no." But this time was different. We'd just returned from a lengthy vacation, where we all were waited on hand and foot. I felt the need to draw a line in the sand. "No sweetheart we can't get her today. Maybe Santa will surprise you at Christmas." Naturally, she was disappointed, but to my delight, took the news pretty well.

As we walked home, I gave some thought to what had just transpired. Saying "no" to someone you love is hard, particularly your kids. But telling a child "no" is a skill, and one that all parents need and should practice without guilt. Lives are at stake.

I shared this story for a reason—we're all in the same boat. Setting limits with children is hard. Many parents indulge their children's every whim. They don't want to live through the discomfort of saying "no" or seeing them unhappy so they just buy them off. But limit setting is a form of self-regulation, teaching kids how to set limits for themselves.

This is a critical, especially if we're to teach our kids about the merits of a heart healthy lifestyle. Eliminating TV, video games, and sugar-sweetened drinks isn't a realistic option for many parents. But restricting their use may help reduce a child's chance of being overweight or obese, prevent future weight gain, and slash their risk of developing diabetes.

We need to teach kids the value of developing the behaviors that lead to a heart-healthy lifestyle. Ideally, it's home, not school that should become the hub of our efforts to ensure that kids take the first steps towards a heart healthy way of living. H-E-A-R-T isn't a random activity. It's self-actualization. Each step is designed to rid the risk factors for heart disease while encouraging behaviors and action most needed to live a heart healthy lifestyle. Working together, we can change course, and improve our children's heart health.

WHAT YOU CAN DO

I tell the parents that treating congenital heart disease is akin to fixing the plumbing or correcting the electrical wiring in their home. Preventing heart disease requires something very different—a change in behavior. As with adults, getting to the root cause of the problem requires a change in behavior.

Medication helps. But of far greater value is changing the behavior that created the need for medication. There's no magic elixir for heart-healthy living. If there were, we'd all be using it. As I've said throughout this book, the problems facing all of us can't be fixed with a pill. With a few notable exceptions, heart disease is a complex behavioral disorder that requires people to make changes. *Pills don't make people change.* The work of H-E-A-R-T is about instilling healthy habits that will last a lifetime.

This has to be a family affair. Every day, I encourage you to remind your children of their H-E-A-R-T and the five most critical steps needed to guard and maintain our most precious organ. Parents, in particular, are in charge of the home environment and this is where it must start.

Remember that achieving a lasting change in behavior starts with a lasting change in thinking. In this regard, kids need our help. Those to whom they're closest and feel the greatest connection shape our children's attitudes and outlook on life. We have to embody the thinking and behavior that will help make the healthiest choice the only choice. At home and at school, we need to motivate and encourage our children to know their numbers and take the steps needed for optimal heart health.

CHAPTER 11

Keeping the Beat: Maintaining Your Heart-Healthy Lifestyle

Now that you're familiar with the model for a heart healthy life, in this concluding chapter, we should finally turn our attention to this book's greatest challenge: Maintenance. Reducing the risk of and ultimately preventing cardiovascular disease involves making major changes. Often, it requires changing the habits and thinking of a lifetime. For years, we've been told to eat less saturated fat, adopt a proper diet, exercise more, monitor our blood pressure, reduce stress, lay off salt, and quit smoking. These are great ideas, of course, but what does it mean to incorporate them into our everyday regimen. "Knowing" what to eat isn't the same thing as doing it and that's the conundrum facing millions looking to prevent or minimize cardiovascular disease and live a heart healthy lifestyle. What stands in our way? What's the obstacle to a life free of heart disease? We are the obstacles. Period. The chasm between "knowing" and "doing" falls squarely at our feet. Thus, this chapter is about closing the gap, teaching us how to think each and every day about our H-E-A-R-T by taking control of our diet, managing our cholesterol and blood pressure, reducing stress, keeping our blood sugar in check, and engaging in some form of daily physical activity. My hope is that after finishing this chapter, H-E-A-R-T is the last prescription you ever receive from a cardiologist.

MARTHA'S STORY

Five days a week the routine always is the same. The alarm clock rings 5:30 AM sharp. But before Martha even gets out of bed, she opens her night table drawer and carefully pulls out a 3 x 5 index card. Inscribed on the card in bold red letters is a single acronym:

H-E-A-R-T. You know the American Express commercial, "Don't leave home without it"? That index card is Martha's constant companion. She doesn't go anywhere without it.

I gave the card to Martha after performing an emergency coronary thrombectomy on her right coronary artery and left main coronary artery, both of which were 94 percent occluded. As its name implies, a coronary thrombectomy is a procedure used to remove a blood clot from the coronary arteries. The RCA and LMCA or *left main trunk* are the two major arteries that supply blood directly to the heart.

At the time of her procedure, Martha was on the downslope of a marriage and estranged from her oldest daughter. She was stuck in a job she despised. By her own conservative estimates, she was 70 pounds overweight, with that weight collecting around hips, thighs and stomach. Anytime she felt like exercising she would lie down until the feeling went away. White potatoes were the only plant food in her diet. She had hypertension, high levels of LDL and triglycerides and low levels of HDL, and her blood sugar was through the roof, and based on the results of her A1C test, which measures blood glucose for the previous two to three months, Martha also was diabetic.

Now, almost two years after her procedure, Martha is a new woman. She's lost 65 pounds, power walks 3 miles a day with arm weights, has adopted a diet that includes ample helpings of heart-healthy fruits and vegetables—except potatoes—and has adopted a deep breathing and meditation practice. Across the board, her numbers are down and she's now in the normal range for blood pressure, blood sugar, cholesterol and triglycerides. She no longer takes any medication, except Plavix to prevent future clots, a statin to stabilize her blood vessels and prevent future plaque rupture and a daily dose of aspirin to prevent heart attacks. Martha and her oldest daughter speak at least once a day, and she became a grandmother for the third time.

Martha knows she dodged a bullet two years ago. She realizes that she was hours away from never seeing her newest grandchild.

She's grateful for this new lease on life. And it's this sense of gratitude that Martha clings to, like a shipwreck survivor holding on to a life preserver. She needs to because when you feel good it's easy to forget. And Martha is in no position to do that.

For the longest time, Martha knew something was up. She was going through tremendous emotional turmoil. She wasn't sleeping well. Her body was betraying her. And it was just a matter of time before the other shoe dropped.

In time, Martha started to experience intermittent chest pain and discomfort.

By the time Martha came to see me the pain in her chest had become almost unbearable. Based on her symptoms and medical condition, I scheduled a coronary angioplasty, an invasive imaging test that would allow me to better see Martha's heart chamber and arteries. Once the clots were found, I used a second, special catheter through her groin into the arteries to aspirate her clots.

Most throbectomy patients are released the following day but given Martha's physical condition, I had her stay three days. It was on the day Martha went home from the hospital that I gave her the index card inscribed with the word H-E-A-R-T.

Five weeks after her procedure, Martha started cardiac rehab. Four mornings a week, she'd do warm up exercises and walk on the treadmill under the direction of a clinical exercise physiologist. Martha was in terrible shape and most mornings it was hard for her to get moving. On those days when she didn't feel like going I reminded Martha to take out her index card and just look at it. "This is your daily reminder. It's your template for living. I know you'd never leave your house without your wallet. From now on, I don't want you to go anywhere without that index card." Usually, I'm not that adamant with patients. But in Martha's case I knew I needed to make an exception.

Almost immediately, Martha lost ten pounds and her outlook improved. Still, it took a while before she started feeling better.

Three months after she started rehab, Martha has dropped another twenty pounds and added an additional day of rehab. She also started walking with friends. By reminding herself every day to follow her H-E-A-R-T, Martha was able to stick with her new exercise regimen. "I'm determined to see this through, Dr. Kennedy. I know the finish line is in sight."

I stopped Martha right there. Though I admired her determination, I had to remind Martha that the work in rehab wasn't a temporary fix. "Martha, I gave you that index card for reason. It should serve as a constantly daily reminder to check your numbers, stick with an exercise plan, eat a heart smart diet and manage your stress. H-E-A-R-T is a lifestyle. You never really arrive. No one does. This is a blueprint for the rest of your life."

Martha got it. She knew I wasn't picking on her. My comments to her were no different than those I share with all of my patients, even those who have no medical problems but just want to know how to prevent heart disease. After twenty years practicing medicine, I'd like to think I understand a bit about human nature. Once the danger has passed, it's easy to forget, to become less vigilant. That can't happen.

Martha's procedure saved her life. But I knew that she'd be right back where she started if she didn't make fundamental changes to the thinking and behavior that landed her on the operating table in the first place. That's why she needed a daily reminder. That's why she needed to follow her H-E-A-R-T.

"I got it, Dr. Kennedy. I'll do anything to prevent this from happening again." Although Martha had been diligent about her rehab and diet, that conversation marked a turning point.

A year after her procedure, Martha was down forty-five pounds and exercising six days a week. She was following the *5 for 1 Diet* and creating gourmet meals and snacks from its hundreds of great tasting, heart healthy foods.

Martha really felt the bad times were behind her but vowed never to let a single day go by without looking at her index card.

Now, twenty-two months after her procedure, Martha is down seventy pounds. She even competed in a five-mile walk race, coming in fifth in her age division. Martha even added swimming and water aerobics to her regimen, hoping to drop another ten pounds to reach her goal weight of 130 pounds.

Looking back, Martha knew how all of this started. But the past is the past. We can't close the barn door after the horses have already escaped. All we can do is move forward.

"This was tough to deal with. And even though I'm feeling better, I know that I can never forget. I need a daily reminder of where I was, where I am now and what I need to do to stay there," she told me.

"Even pain wasn't motivation enough. I now know it's easier to prevent than to repeat it. But only be able to do this if I follow my H-E-A-R-T."

THE GREAT MOTIVATOR... OR NOT

Pain is a great motivator. If you've ever experienced an abscessed tooth, bad back, migraine headache, shingles, or even a frozen shoulder then you'll identify immediately with that sentiment. Think about it. Take lower back pain for an example. You'll do anything—take a hot path, down some ibuprofen, visit the chiropractor, sleep on a wooden board, visit a shaman, light a candle to Saint Peter, endure a cortisol injection, and even go under the knife—to find some relief.

Hands down, pain is the one symptom that brings more people to my office than all other symptoms combined. It provides you with structure and gives focus. Pain motivates people to make an appointment. Pain motivates people off their couches and into my office. Pain is the impetus that forces them to do something about their situation. Pain is the primary motivation for the most significant changes we make in our lives.

Pain is our body's call to arms. By design, the loudest alarm—the pain we cannot ignore—is the pain saved for last. Pain gets our attention and persists until we do something to help the situation. It is designed to motivate us into action.

Pain can be a good thing. There's no growth without pain, hence the expression "growing pain." Too often, pain is viewed as the problem. Pain is information. With heart disease, it's the body's loudest alarm and the motivation to make changes.

It may seem odd for me to say this but pain also is the great pretender. Pain sticks around for as long as we need it but once the crisis passes, so does the pain. This is normal. We distance ourselves from the experience of pain. How could we move forward otherwise?

SKIPPING A BEAT: WHY SOME PEOPLE FLUNK H-E-A-R-T

Health crises motivate us to change. Who wouldn't be motivated by the thought of dying prematurely or severe disability? Imagine that you've been diagnosed with secondary hypertension, meaning your hypertension has a definite cause such as obesity, kidney disease or thyroid disorder. Right away, you spring into action. You follow your doctor's advice to the letter of the law. You keep to a strict diet, rest, watch your stress, and check your numbers. You take your medication. You recruit the support of family and friends to help you make it through this latest crisis.

Three months go by and you reach your destination. Your pressure has stabilized. You look and feel much better. Most importantly, your health has improved. You'd think this would be motivation enough to hold on to your hard earned gains. But as Daniel Ariely, the James B. Duke Professor of Psychology and Behavioral Economics at Duke University, observes in his *New York Times* bestseller, *Predictably Irrational: The Hidden Forces That Shape Our Decisions*, seldom do people behave rationally when it comes to making important, real-life decisions. Human behavior is seldom about what's rational. It is, as Professor Ariely says, "predictably irrational."[1]

Human behavior is the logic of the psyche, which is *psycho*logic, and not really logic at all. This is the logic of the moment. It's "feel good" logic—it's the logic of our emotions and feelings. To quote a line from a favorite yoga teacher, "Have your feelings, just don't buy them." Feelings often get the best of us.

How do you *keep the beat?* What are the secrets to maintaining a heart-healthy lifestyle after the obvious motivation—your health crisis—is no longer there? How do you cope when friends and family who were there while you dealt with this latest health crisis, stop coming around. Where's the incentive to keep going once you need to see the doctor less frequently?

Taking it a step further, how to stay vigilant if you don't have any risk factors or have never even had heart disease?

The classic disease model suggests that there is a beginning, middle and end to a problem. This is especially true for acute conditions like appendicitis or an aneurysm. But there is no end game when it comes to reversing and preventing heart disease. It's a lifelong endeavor. By and large, heart disease is a chronic illness. There's a reason for this. The disease model pays too little attention to the behavioral component of heart disease. You can't just heal your hypertension, reduce your blood sugar and tackle your triglycerides and suddenly think that everything is OK. What is it about your thinking that caused you to have high blood pressure and blood sugar and elevated cholesterol? The real changes occur when you embody the thinking and behavior needed to *keep the beat*.

Some people who *skip a beat* lose structure. And what is the disease treatment paradigm but a structured way of doing things. Health crises provide you with structure. They sharpen your focus. But once the danger passes, you may feel that it's OK to ease up on the pedal. Maybe you stop checking your numbers, have a few extra cookies or second helping of ice cream, stop exercising, and don't look for healthy outlets for stress.

Two years ago, a former patient came to see me. I performed a coronary angioplasty on her when I was a cardiology fellow in San Francisco. At the time of her procedure, she was fifty pounds overweight, her daily exercise routine consisted of opening and closing the refrigerator door and she had severely elevated LDL cholesterol and triglycerides, among many other health concerns. When I saw her again nearly eighteen years later, I was delighted to see that at age seventy-two she was still following the healthy heart template I designed for her. In doing so, she was able to reverse her medical condition and eliminate all of her risk factors, and even prevent future recurrences. H-E-A-R-T gave my patient the structure most chronic disease patients need but sorely lack.

Once your health improves, H-E-A-R-T is still in place. If you've never had heart disease or have known risk factors and are just looking to *keep the beat,* H-E-A-R-T still applies. *People who succeed at reversing and preventing heart disease practice* **vigilance**—*the number one strategy for obtaining and maintaining optimal heart health.*

Even people who achieve all five numbers still fall back into old patterns of behavior. They've healed their hypertension, energized their bodies, attacked their adipose, reduced their blood sugar, and

THE FIVE TOP REASONS WHY WE *SKIP A BEAT*

No matter how much resolve you think you may have, keeping the beat and maintaining a H-E-A-R-T healthy lifestyle isn't easy. There are forces at work, most notably maladaptive thinking and behavior that can weaken your resolve and challenge you to maintain your hard earned gains.

1. We have too much to do with too little time to do it.
2. We have no time to exercise.
3. We don't have time to eat right or to make healthy food choices.
4. We ignore stress in our life and attempt to self-medicate with maladaptive behaviors like smoking, drinking, and overeating.
5. We ignore the daily vicious cycle. Difficult commute, challenging workplace, commute home, home stress, poor sleep, difficult morning commute back to work.

tackled their triglycerides and cholesterol. This took work. What's wrong with celebrating a little? Well, if you could celebrate a *little* that would be fine. But all evidence points to the contrary. Who wants to do a "little" of something that feels good? *Be careful with starting with a little. It could end up costing you a lot.*

KEEPING THE BEAT: WINNING H-E-A-R-T

With any prevention model, what you do for yourself is going to have a much greater impact on your long-term well-being than anything I can do for you medically, particularly in the context of an office visit. Even the most complex and invasive surgical procedure has an end point. If you need medication I'll prescribe it. If I have to unclog a blocked artery and put in a stent, I will do that. But what's next?

Think about the example of the recovering drug addict. After physical detox, most often done under careful medical supervision, many addicts turn to support groups like 12-step recovery. There's nothing random about this. We now know that 12-step recovery isn't something people just do for fun or to pass the time. In fact, there's nothing random about 12-step recovery. It's actually a complex neurophysiological process that literally reshapes the brain, helping free people from self-destructive behavior, and maladaptive thinking that first led them to abuse drugs.

Recovering from hypertension, pre-diabetes or even type 2 diabetes is no different. Once the symptoms have been treated, what steps do we put in place that treat the behavior that caused these risk factors to surface?

To start, set a goal and be specific. Using H-E-A-R-T as a template, think of something you can do every day to reverse or prevent hypertension, attack fat, reduce blood sugar, and tackle your triglycerides and cholesterol. Take the "E" in H-E-A-R-T and commit every day to walk thirty minutes a day for a week. Notice I say, "walk thirty minutes a day" and not "commit to physical activity." The more specific, the more likely you are to stick with your plan. Also, keep things simple. Having too many goals can feel overwhelming and have the opposite effect of eroding your motivation and resolve.

The other critical thing to remember is that H-E-A-R-T isn't a quick fix. This isn't a test just to determine your risk of a coronary event. Rather, H-E-A-R-T is a lifestyle. And maintenance is most critical component of that lifestyle.

Maintenance will always challenge you. You'll always be thinking, "What's next?" That's why you need H-E-A-R-T. Willpower or strength of character alone won't save you. If that were true, then heart disease wouldn't be the number one cause of death for men and women in the United States. You need a plan. You need strategies. And the number one strategy is a change in the thinking and behavior that caused your problems in the first place. Without a change in thinking, you'll just end up right back where you started.

To keep the beat and succeed at H-E-A-R-T you must remember that the journey is the destination. You don't ever arrive at perfect heart health. Why? With any chronic disease you don't ever completely lose your vulnerability. Just because you've lost thirty pounds, exercise regularly, and have achieved great numbers for cholesterol and blood sugar doesn't mean you're any different than the guy who sat in my office a few years ago with pre-metabolic syndrome. If you're like millions of heart patients, you have the same personality, the same eating style and the same disdain for exercise. H-E-A-R-T isn't the equivalent of winning a 10K race. Achieving an ideal weight, exercising, and managing your stress means that battle has just begun.

BREAKING THE CYCLE: JOEY'S STORY

Joey got used to being without his dad. As one of three kids in a military family, Joey's father, a Marine Corporal, was away more than he was home. Career military men, "lifers," as they're called, are at the government's beckon call, and frequently find themselves in far flung destinations, often at their family's expense.

When Joey's dad was home he'd tried to make up for lost time. Ball games, amusement parks, weekend camping trips, and day trips to beach were just a few of things he loved to do with his kids. On the other hand, Joey's dad also believed his kids should toe the line and was not beyond making sure the message hit home with a belt or back of the hand. "Another way of making up for lost time," his frustrated wife would complain to friends.

Joey tried to be good. He certainly didn't want to catch a spanking or slap across the face, especially after not seeing his dad for nearly six months. But no kid is perfect, especially a rambunctious four-year-old who loved nothing more than climbing trees, wading through streams looking for crayfish, and tagging along with his older siblings as they bounced from one activity to another.

The problem for Joey, as well as his brother and sister, is that he never knew what would set the old man off. It could be something seemingly innocuous like the time Joey and his older brother, Tim, accidentally landed in their mother's flowerbed while riding their scooters in the driveway. Or, the time when Joey tore a hole in his new shirt while climbing over the backyard fence. "You're gonna pay holy hell for that one," his dad said after learning of the torn shirt. Joey knew what was coming.

The other thing with military families is that they move a lot. The family was constantly on the go. Most military families move every two to three years. The family accepted this reality, but the frequent upheavals were difficult, especially for the kids. As the youngest, Joey seemed to have the most difficult time transitioning from one place to the next. He didn't complain, of course. He didn't want to incur the old man's wrath.

After three years, and three moves, including one across the country, Joey's dad announced to the family that he'd been given a desk job and would be home for a while. Moreover, the family would be staying at their current location, and wouldn't be moving for the foreseeable future. They settled into a comfortable home, at least by military standards, in a quiet suburban neighborhood about twenty miles east of Los Angeles. There was a big backyard with lots of trees and even space for a swimming pool and small vegetable garden. Joey loved climbing the trees, as did his brother and sister. The three siblings talked about building a tree house and forming a special "members only" club. Problem is that Joey's father, who seemed to be settling in nicely to life in Southern California, didn't love his kids nonstop climbing. In fact, he expressly forbade them from climbing the trees. "They're young. I don't want them to get hurt. I'm not going to allow it," he told his wife, who seemed bewildered by her husband's concerns, but nevertheless went along, as she always did, with his latest edict.

But Joey loved climbing the backyard trees, more so than his older siblings. From a favorite perch high above the lawn, he'd survey the neighborhood landscape. He was especially fascinated with the telephone repairmen. He'd spend hours watching them, tools in hand as they went up and down the utility poles. He fanaticized about becoming a repairman. As they'd scale the utility poles, he'd climb his favorite tree, copying their every move. Unbeknownst to his father, Joey's mother even brought him a toy tool belt so he could work alongside the repairmen. He'd share stories of the repairmen's exploits with his mother, amusing her with talk about his career goals.

After several months of relative tranquility, Joey's father announced over dinner that he'd be leaving for a second tour of Far East Asia. Things had been going well and everyone was upset by the news, especially Joey, who seemed hard hit by his father's sudden announcement.

After his father left, Joey spent even more time up the tree on his favorite branch watching the telephone repairmen. In the distance, Joey hears his mother voice calling him to help set the table. He started climbing down from the tree, just as he'd done a hundred times in the past year. As Joey was lowering his foot to the branch closest to the ground, he loses his grip, and comes crashing down, landing awkwardly on his left arm. Joey's mom, who's preparing dinner, hears her youngest son's anguished cries and comes running. She sees him lying beside the tree, holding his left arm with his right hand. It's clear to her that Joey has broken his arm. Just as she bends down to pick up Joey, he blurts out, "Daddy's going to be upset. He told me not to climb the tree. He's going to spank me when he gets home."

Turns out, Joey's father was gone longer than expected and Joey's mother, who worried about her son incurring her husband's wrath, never told him how Joey broke his arm. It's never a good idea to lie, but in this case, discretion seemed the better part of valor.

Years passed, and Joey grew into a fine young man, even realizing his childhood dream of becoming a telephone repairman. Joey's father had long since died of a heart attack triggered by advanced atherosclerosis, which he'd ignored until it was too late. Joey loved his life and work. He even imagined his own son following in his footsteps someday.

Early one morning, Joey started his work as he always does: Climbing up a utility pole. It was warm, but not unusually so. But since his job offered little protection from the elements, Joey always made sure to take precautions on warm days, drinking plenty of water, especially if he knew that he'd working outside.

Just as he reached the top of the utility pole Joey felt a sharp pain in his chest. "Indigestion," was his first thought since he'd treated himself to a second helping of his wife's vegetarian pasta the night before. But Joey soon realized this was no ordinary case of indigestion. Indeed, the pain, which has been confined to his chest, started radiating up is jaw, back and down his left arm. Quickly, he climbed down the utility pole. Funny thing, as soon as Joey touched down he started feeling better. "Panic attack," he thought to himself. Still, Joey scheduled an appointment with his internist. Why take risks? He had a family to support.

As Joey discussed his symptoms the following day, sharing that he'd been experiencing them with greater frequency and always when he climbed a utility pole. His doctor suspected something more and sent him to me. I sent Joey for exercise cardiac stress testing (ECST) and the most widely used cardiac stress test. This is a test where a patient runs on a treadmill while his electrocardiogram (EKG), heart rate, heart rhythm, and blood pressure are continuously monitored. If a coronary arterial blockage results in decreased blood flow to a part of the heart during exercise, certain changes may be observed in the EKG, as well as in the response of the heart rate and blood pressure. The tests results led me to believe that Joey had CAD, which was confirmed with angiogram and followed up with a stent to improve blood flow to his blocked coronary artery.

Joey returned to work six weeks after his procedure. Still, he was worried. The minute he started climbing the pole that same panicky feeling set in. This time, there could be no issue with his heart. Joey called me the following day and I suggested he contact a therapist. It's during therapy that Joey finally discovers the root of his ongoing anxiety. Joey still associates climbing the utility pole with the beatings he received from his father when he climbed a tree. Almost three decades have elapsed but he's still reliving that traumatic event. The therapist told Joey he was suffering from post-traumatic stress disorder (PTSD), which very likely contributed to his atherosclerosis since he didn't have any other obvious risk factors. Indeed, people with PTSD may be at increased risk of heart attacks and strokes. "PTSD doesn't just impact your head. It harms your body," said Joey's therapist.

Suddenly, all the pieces started falling into place. Joey realized that his dad, a two-toured Vietnam veteran, also suffered from PTSD, which was no doubt triggered by the horror of combat. Sadly, he developed maladaptive behavior for dealing with his condition. "Physical abuse, especially during childhood, can also trigger PTSD," confirmed Joey's therapist.

While there's no direct evidence correlating PTSD and heart disease, it's not coincidental that sufferers smoke, and have high rates or alcoholism and hypertension, which could contribute to heart disease risks. Imaging studies of the hearts of people with PTSD have shown decreased blood flow, which no doubt stem from stress-induced lifestyle choices..

After just a month of therapy, Joey's panic attacks begin to subside. It was the combined therapy of fixing his arteries and head that set Joey on the path to cardiovascular health. Joey even returned to his job with renewed confidence and sense of purpose. Both Joey and his wife committed themselves to "breaking the cycle," and doing everything humanly possible to keep heart disease from again touching their lives.

Joey even imparted the wisdom from lessons learned to his kids, enrolling them in yoga classes, teaching them to be present and helping them find creative and healthy outlets for stress.

Each of my patients' personal stories resonates with me. They are my greatest teachers and I learn as much, if not more from them as they do from me. They've created many of the techniques and strategies I share with you in the HEART HEALTH BIBLE. But Joey's is different. On the deepest level, it's an embrace of this book's prevention message. Joey was born into a family with a legacy of heart disease. But that legacy wasn't a life sentence. Using H-E-A-R-T, Joey was able to change course.

Joey's story also brought up an age-old medical tautology: Did coronary artery disease develop first? Or, did the repeated stress of climbing the telephone pole and the unconscious conflicts it triggered bring on the disease? Joey wasn't even aware of the family legacy until he came to see me.

In some ways the old chicken and egg argument is a non sequitur. Joey's story teaches us that our thinking and feelings affect heart disease. And the point to make is that Joey grabbed the ball of his tragic family legacy and ran in the opposite direction. He was determined that the specter of heart disease wouldn't hover over his family. He taught his kids the value of eating right, exercise and stress management. He gave them the tools they'd need to manage the slings and arrows of life's misfortunes.

In life, the apple doesn't fall far from the tree. But Joey's awareness triggered a paradigm shift in thinking. Joey's insight about his father and how it affected his own physical and emotional well-being proved to be a revelation, completely redirecting his approach to living. Without this insight, the cycle may have continued. Joey wouldn't allow that. He gave his kids the tools. He gave them H-E-A-R-T—the new family legacy.

H-E-A-R-T: YOUR PERSONAL PREVENTION PORTFOLIO

Picture this: You're sixty-three. Retirement is just a short fourteen months away after nearly four decades of work. Right out of college, you hit the ground running, clawing your way up the corporate ranks to your current position of Senior Vice President. You and Judy have been married for thirty-eight years and successfully put three kids through college. You own two homes outright and property in three different states. You've invested wisely and saved prudently. You've traveled the world multiple times. Your retirement nest egg has been incubating for years.

Five years ago everything changed. Your stocks crashed, the real estate market nosedived. Like millions of other people, you took a huge hit, losing nearly 45 percent of your retirement savings and watching your property values drop sharply. Suddenly, retirement no longer seems like a viable option. You decide to put things off for a couple of years, assuming the economy will turn around.

This couple, both my patients, did everything by the book. But they couldn't foresee a game changing market decline and global economic crisis. No one could. We can't predict the future. That's why we need a plan in place.

But financial planning is not a do-it-yourself endeavor. In our modern world, there are myriad tools available to help us to manage our money: online tax preparers, online stock trading, online mortgage calculators, online investment advisors, and online insurance brokers. If you could have an online cardiologist available at your beckon call, would you still take matters into your own hands? Of course you wouldn't. Brakes stall? Call a mechanic. Annoying toothache? Visit the dentist.

You have to consistently invest to plan for and maintain a sound financial future. Just as stocks and bonds can be an investment in your financial future, H-E-A-R-T is an investment in your health. It's a daily investment in your health.

That doesn't mean you're home free. We can't control the global markets. We can't control everything that happens to us. But H-E-A-R-T is reassurance, something to always fall back on. Unlike financial markets where there's an accepted concept of risk/reward, you don't want to play Russian roulette with your health. We can take risks with our finances. Taking a risk with H-E-A-R-T always yields a bad outcome.

All of us have dreams about what we want out of life. For many, the goal of achieving a comfortable lifestyle starts by building a financial portfolio, complete with well-funded retirement accounts, emergency cash reserve, and diversified investments. In the same way that you set up a financial portfolio to plan for the future, you need to establish your personal prevention portfolio to achieve your goal of a heart healthy future. It's one thing to lose weight and lower your blood pressure. It's another matter to maintain those hard won goals. Using the template of the five steps, I'd ask you to consider a brand new script—a heart health road map—to help you develop a personalized cardiovascular disease prevention plan. Ultimately, this new script is about freedom, giving rise to a deep confidence in your ability to take control of your cardiovascular health and make the great leap forward into a new era of wellness.

Epilogue

YOUR MORNING ROUNDS

Each morning I start my daily cardiology rounds on patients admitted to various hospitals all around the Los Angeles area. Some are critically ill and are admitted to the intensive care units where they recover from recent cardiovascular events. On each of the patients, I feel and record their pulse and vital signs and I am constantly reminded of how most of us ignore our heart until sometimes it is too late, which makes me wonder as I write orders for medications and tests whether these hospitalizations could have been avoided if they had only followed their H-E-A-R-T.

If they had only committed to the information in this book and periodically checked their pulse, maybe this hospitalization could have been avoided. Although most of the risk factors for heart disease, like high blood pressure, physical inactivity, increased waist size, elevated blood sugar, and high cholesterol occur in most without symptoms, it is important to always be aware of and follow your H-E-A-R-T. Our heart, although quiet and unassuming, is our most vital and precious organ and for optimal performance requires maintenance and attention and reminds me of the quote:

Let your heart guide you. It whispers, so listen closely....Land Before Time.

And once you have achieved your 5 numbers make sure you share this life saving knowledge with a loved one, family member and friend because as John Andrew Holmes once said: A good exercise for the heart is to bend down and help another up....

John

ABOUT THE AUTHOR

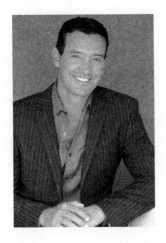

Dr. John M. Kennedy is a recognized expert in the field of invasive cardiology and a much sought after authority on complimentary medical approaches. He has successfully helped thousands of patients with his pioneering to preventive cardiology since beginning his practice 20 years ago. Board-certified in internal medicine, cardiovascular disease, board member of the American Heart Association and a clinical associate professor of cardiology at Harbor-UCLA Medical Center, Dr. Kennedy is a dedicated healer who approaches the business of 'health' with compassion, intention, and commitment. He believes that the seeds needed to reverse and ultimately prevent heart disease reside in all of us, but must be cultivated and nurtured with mindful, dedicated time and attention. Dr. Kennedy's approach to heart health is consultative and instructive, not prescriptive. He would much prefer that you change your diet and learn to manage your stress than put in a stent or perform cardiac catheterization. And while he believes you can transcend cardiovascular disease with lifestyle modification, there is no "magic formula (bullet)" that works for everyone. The results are proportional to the work and mindfulness to a person's efforts. His deeply rooted belief that everyone has an inner potential for greater heart health is the foundation on which he now bases his practice of preventive cardiology and wellness.

Dr. Kennedy is a Director of Preventive Cardiology and Wellness at Marina Del Rey Hospital. His program specializes in rehabilitation, early detection and the treatment of cardiac problems, with an emphasis on prevention. Based on a large body of literature showing how stress adversely impacts heart health, as well as his own cutting-edge research on post-stroke patients, Dr. Kennedy created the BREATHE™ technique to stop stress in its tracks. By combining two time-honored forms of relaxation - guided imagery and breath work - Dr. Kennedy has created a new paradigm in stress management, which an ABC News investigative story concluded, "could reduce high blood pressure in as little as two weeks."

Along with his work in the field of preventive cardiology, Dr. Kennedy is an integral part of the team at LA Bariatrics. Dr. Kennedy encourages patients to adopt and maintain new, healthier lifestyle habits so they not only lose weight but also, more importantly, keep it off.

The media and health industry luminaries frequently turn to Dr. Kennedy as a resource for information on preventive cardiology and wellness. Dr. Kennedy has appeared on the internationally syndicated CBS show *The Doctors* and has been featured on *The Dr. Oz Show*, *World News with Diane Sawyer*, *Anderson Cooper*, *Katie* and PBS. He has appeared in print media in *First for Women*, *The Advocate*, *Health Magazine*, *Real Simple Magazine*, *The Guardian* and online in MSN's Today Health, Everyday Health. In his quest to bring knowledge to the public, he hosts MD-VOD, a live show that provides simple answers to common medical questions and problems. He also lectures throughout the United States and holds regular seminars on cardiovascular disease, stress management, healthy nutrition and dieting, proper breathing, and more. Recognizing the growing prevalence of heart disease among children, Dr. Kennedy also has made it his personal crusade to educate children about the importance of diet, exercise and stress management in his popular talk entitled, Big Mind, Brave Heart, Bright Future.

Dr. Kennedy's first book for popular audiences, the critically acclaimed *The 15 Minute Heart Cure: The Natural Way to Release Stress and Heal Your Heart in Just Minutes a Day*, was hailed by Ralph Brindis, M.D., President, American College of Cardiology, as "an outstanding review of a timely and important subject, stress and heart disease." Visit Dr. Kennedy's website to learn more about the BREATHE™ Technique.

In 2012, Dr. Kennedy co-founded Encardea (http://encardea. com/index.htm), a one-of-a-kind wellness company offering interactive applications and websites, books and multi-media tools to foster a heightened and enlightened awareness of the necessary steps to cope with the challenges of everyday life, including depression, anxiety, loss, disease, smoking, weight management, high blood pressure, work-related stress, anger, bullying, parenting and more.

Prior to his appointment as director of preventative cardiology and wellness at Marina Del Rey Hospital, Dr. Kennedy was director of the cardiac catheterization lab at Kaiser Permanente in San Rafael California, where he created the Heart Alert Program—the gold standard nationwide for rapidly and effectively treating heart attack patients. Dr. Kennedy also was the co-director of the cardiac CT angiography program at Kaiser Permanente. His cutting-edge research in the fields of cardiac calcification and cardiac imaging has been published in numerous peer-reviewed journals including the Journal of the American College of Cardiology. Year after year, Dr.

Kennedy finds his name included in Castle Connolly's list of the nation's top cardiologists. Dr. Kennedy received his medical degree from the Dartmouth-Brown Program in Medicine and his B.S. from the University of California-Santa Barbara, from which he graduated summa cum laude. He holds membership in several professional medical organizations, including The American College of Cardiology. His numerous awards and honors include election to the prestigious Sigma Xi Scientific Research Society. Dr. Kennedy currently resides in Los Angeles, California.

REFERENCES AND FURTHER READING

The data and findings discovered in this work serve as the founda-tion and everlasting evidence supporting the importance of following your H-E-A-R-T.

THE HEART OF THE MATTER: METABOLIC SYNDROME

Scott M. Grundy et al. Diagnosis and Management of the Metabolic Syn-drome, An American Heart Association/National Heart, Lung, and Blood Institute Scientific Statement: Executive Summary.

Isomaa B, Almgren P, Tuomi T. et al. Cardiovascular morbidity and mortal-ity associated with the metabolic syndrome. Diabetes Care. 2001; 24:683–689.

National Institutes of Health. Third Report of the National Cholesterol Education Program Expert Panel on Detection, Evaluation, and Treat-ment of High Blood Cholesterol in Adults (Adult Treatment Panel III). Bethesda, Md: National Institutes of Health; 2001. NIH Publica-tion 01–3670.

LEARN 5 NOW AND PREVENT 5 LATER: KIDS AND HEART DISEASE

American Academy of Pediatrics. Cardiovascular risk reduction in high-risk pediatric populations. Pediatrics 2007; 119:618.

Kavey RE, Allada V, Daniels SR, et al. Cardiovascular risk reduction in high-risk pediatric patients: a scientific statement from the American Heart Association Expert Panel on Population and Prevention Science; the Councils on Cardiovascular Disease in the Young, Epidemiology and Prevention, Nutrition, Physical Activity and Metabolism, High Blood Pressure Research, Cardiovascular Nursing, and the Kidney in Heart Disease; and the Interdisciplinary Working Group on Quality of Care and Outcomes Research: endorsed by the American Academy of Pediatrics. Circulation 2006; 114:2710.

Berenson GS, Srinivasan SR, Bao W, et al. Association between multiple cardiovascular risk factors and atherosclerosis in children and young adults. The Bogalusa Heart Study. N Engl J Med 1998; 338:1650.

H—HEAL YOUR BLOOD PRESSURE

Kearney PM, Whelton M, Reynolds K, et al. Global burden of hypertension: analysis of worldwide data. Lancet. 2005; 365(9455):217–223.

Walley T, Duggan AK, Haycox AR, Niziol CJ. Treatment for newly diagnosed hypertension: patterns of prescribing and antihypertensive effectiveness in the UK. J R Soc Med. 2003; 96(11):525–531.

Heagerty A. Optimizing hypertension management in clinical practice. J Hum Hypertens. 2006; 20(11):841–849.

Department of Health. Statistics for General Medical Practitioners in England: 1994–2004. London: Department of Health, 2005.

Sacks FM, Svetkey LP, Vollmer WM, et al. Effects on blood pressure of reduced dietary sodium and the Dietary Approaches to Stop Hypertension (DASH) diet. DASH-Sodium Collaborative Research Group. N Engl J Med. 2001; 344(1):3–10.

E—ENERGIZE AND EXERCISE FOR A HEALTHY HEART

Berry JD, Willis B, Gupta S, et al. Lifetime risks for cardiovascular disease mortality by cardiorespiratory fitness levels measured at ages 45, 55, and 65 years in men the cooper center longitudinal study. J Am Coll Cardiol. Apr 12 2011; 57(15):1604-10.

Wen CP, Wai JP, Tsai MK, et al. Minimum amount of physical activity for reduced mortality and extended life expectancy: a prospective cohort study. Lancet. Oct 1 2011; 378(9798):1244–53 [Medline].

Artinian NT, Fletcher GF, Mozaffarian D, Kris-Etherton P, Van Horn L, Lichtenstein AH, et al. Interventions to promote physical activity and dietary lifestyle changes for cardiovascular risk factor reduction in adults: a scientific statement from the American Heart Association. Circulation. Jul 27 2010; 122(4):406–41 [Medline].

Rana JS, Arsenault BJ, Després JP, Côté M, Talmud PJ, Ninio E, et al. Inflammatory biomarkers, physical activity, waist circumference, and risk of future coronary heart disease in healthy men and women. Eur Heart J. Feb 2011; 32(3):336–44.

A—ACT ON FAT: OBESITY

Institute of Medicine. Accelerating progress in obesity prevention: solving the weight of the nation. Washington, DC: National Academies Press; 2012. Available at: www.iom.edu/Reports/2012/Accelerating-Progress-in-Obesity-Prevention.aspx. Accessed January 18, 2012.

Wang Y, Lobstein TM. Worldwide trends in childhood overweight and obesity. Int Journal of Pediatric Obesity. 2006; 1(1):11–25.

Wang Y, Beydoun MA. The obesity epidemic in the United States—gender, age, socioeconomic, racial/ethnic, and geographic characteristics: a systematic review and meta-regression analysis. Epidemiol Rev. 2007; 29(1):6–28pmid:17510091.

Ogden CL, Carroll MD, Kit BK, Flegal KM. Prevalence of obesity and trends in body mass index among US children and adolescents, 1999-2010. JAMA. 2012; 307(5):483–490pmid:22253364.

Whitaker RC, Wright JA, Pepe MS, Seidel KD, Dietz WH. Predicting obesity in young adulthood from childhood and parental obesity. N Engl J Med. 1997; 337(13):869–873pmid:9302300.

Strauss RS. Childhood obesity and self-esteem. Pediatrics. 2000; 105(1). Available at: www.pediatrics.org/cgi/content/full/

Golan M. Parents as agents of change in childhood obesity—from research to practice. Int J Pediatr Obes. 2006;1(2):66–76pmid:17907317.

Birch LL, Davison KK. Family environmental factors influencing the developing behavioral controls of food intake and childhood overweight. Pediatr Clin North Am. 2001;48(4):893–907pmid:11494642.

Gerards SM, Sleddens EF, Dagnelie PC, et al. Intervention addressing general parenting to prevent or treat childhood obesity. Int J Pediatr Obes. 2011;6(2-2):e28–e45.

Wang Y, Wu Y, Wilson RF, et al. Childhood Obesity Prevention Programs: A Comparative Effectiveness Review and Meta-analysis. (Prepared by The Johns Hopkins University Evidence-based Practice Center under contract HHSA-290-2007-10061-I). Rockville, MD: Agency for Healthcare Research and Quality, 2013.

Epstein LH, Gordy CC, Raynor HA, et al. Increasing fruit and vegetable intake and decreasing fat and sugar intake in families at risk for childhood obesity. Obes Res. 2001; 9 (3):171–178.

Patrick K, Calfas KJ, Norman GJ, et al, Randomized controlled trial of a primary care and home-based intervention for physical activity and nutrition behaviors: PACE+ for adolescents. Arch Pediatr Adolesc Med. 2006; 160(2):128–136pmid:16461867.

Brotman LM, Dawson-McClure S, et al. Early childhood family intervention and long-term obesity prevention among high-risk minority youth. Pediatrics.2012; 129(3).

R—REDUCE YOUR BLOOD SUGAR AND DIABETES

Joint Guideline on Intensive Glycemic Control and the Prevention of Cardiovascular Events, LIZ HORSLEY, Am Fam Physician. 2009 Nov 15; 80(10):1167–1170.

Mechanick JI, Camacho PM, Cobin RH, et al; American Association of Clinical Endocrinologists. American Association of Clinical Endocrinologists Protocol for Standardized Production of Clinical Practice Guidelines—2010 update. Endocr Pract. 2010;16:270-283. EL 4; CPG NE; see Figure 1; Table 1-4.

Garber AJ, Handelsman Y, Einhorn D, et al. Diagnosis and management of prediabetes in the continuum of hyperglycemia: When do the risks of diabetes begin? A consensus statement from the American College of Endocrinology and the American Association of Clinical Endocrinologists. Endocr Pract. 2008; 14:933–946.

Moghissi ES, Korytkowski MT, DiNardo M, et al American Association of Clinical Endocrinologists; American Diabetes Association. American Association of Clinical Endocrinologists and American Diabetes Association consensus statement on inpatient glycemic control. Endocr Pract. 2009;15:353-369.

Torgerson JS, Hauptman J, Boldrin MN, Sjöström L. XENical in the prevention of diabetes in obese subjects (XENDOS) study: A randomized study of orlistat as an adjunct to lifestyle changes for the prevention of type 2 diabetes in obese patients [Erratum in Diabetes Care. 2004;27:856]. Diabetes Care. 2004; 27:155-161.

Knowler WC, Barrett-Connor E, Fowler SE, et al; Diabetes Prevention Program Research Group. Reduction in the incidence of type 2 diabetes with lifestyle intervention or metformin. N Engl J Med. 2002; 346:393-403.

Chiasson JL, Josse RG, Gomis R, Hanefeld M, Karasik A, Laakso M; STOP-NIDDM Trial Research Group. Acarbose treatment and the risk of cardiovascular disease and hypertension in patients with impaired glucose tolerance: the STOP-NIDDM trial. JAMA. 2003; 290:486-494.

Chiasson JL, Josse RG, Gomis R, Hanefeld M, Karasik A, Laakso M; STOP-NIDDM Trial Research Group. Acarbose for the prevention of Type 2 diabetes, hypertension and cardiovascular disease in subjects with impaired glucose tolerance: Facts and interpretations concerning the critical analysis of the STOP-NIDDM Trial data. Diabetologia. 2004; 47:969-975.

DREAM (Diabetes REduction Assessment with ramipril and rosiglitazone Medication) Trial Investigators, Gerstein HC, Yusuf S, et al. Effect of rosiglitazone on the frequency of diabetes in patients with impaired glucose tolerance or impaired fasting glucose: A randomised controlled trial [Erratum in: Lancet. 2006; 368:1770].

Defronzo RA, Banerji M, Bray GA, et al. Actos Now for the prevention of diabetes (ACT NOW) study. BMC Endocr Disord. 2009; 9:17.

T—TACKLE TRIGLYCERIDES: CHOLESTEROL

Third Report of the Expert Panel on Detection, Evaluation, and Treatment of High Blood Cholesterol in Adults (ATP III Final Report), Third Report of the Expert Panel on Detection, Evaluation, and Treatment of High Blood Cholesterol in Adults (Adult Treatment Panel III, or ATP III) presents the National Cholesterol Education Program (NCEP) updated recommendations on cholesterol testing and management. The ATP III document is an evidence-based report that provides the scientific rationale for the recommendations contained in the Executive Summary.

The Adult Treatment Panel III (ATP III) of the National Cholesterol Education Program issued an evidence-based set of guidelines on cholesterol management in 2001 (Executive Summary published in JAMA, 2001; 285:2486-2497). Since the publication of ATP III, 5 major clinical trials of statin therapy with clinical end points have been published. These trials addressed issues that were not examined in previous clinical trials of choles-terol-lowering therapy. The present document reviews the results of these recent trials and assesses their implications for cholesterol management.

Executive summary of the Third Report of the National Cholesterol Educa-tion Program (NCEP) Expert Panel on Detection, Evaluation, and Treat-ment of High Blood Cholesterol in Adults (Adult Treatment Panel III).. JAMA. 2001; 285:2486–97.

Lewis SJ, Moye LA, Sacks FM, Johnstone DE, Timmis G, Mitchell J, et al. Effect of pravastatin on cardiovascular events in older patients with myo-cardial infarction and cholesterol levels in the average range. Results of the Cholesterol and Recurrent Events (CARE) trial. Ann Intern Med. 1998;129:681–9.

Berlin JA, Colditz GA. A meta-analysis of physical activity in the preven-tion of coronary heart disease. Am J Epidemiol. 1990; 132:612–28.

Safeer RS, Lacivita CL. Choosing drug therapy for patients with hyperlipi-demia. Am Fam Physician. 2000;61:3371–82.

Rao G. Insulin resistance syndrome. Am Fam Physician. 2001; 63:1159–63.1165–6.

Garg A. Insulin resistance in the pathogenesis of dyslipidemia. Diabetes Care. 1996;19:387–9.

PRIMARY & Secondary Prevention—CAD 48. Lifestyle Heart Trial: Or-nish, et al. Lancet. http://www.ornishspectrum.com/wp-content/uploads/Intensive-lifestyle-changes-for-reversal-of-coronary-heart-disease1.pdf

Smith SC, Jr., Allen J, Blair SN, et al. AHA/ACC guidelines for secondary prevention for patients with coronary and other atherosclerotic vascular disease: 2006 update: endorsed by the National Heart, Lung, and Blood Institute. Circulation 2006; 113:2363–72.

Smith SC, Benjamin EJ, Bonow RO, et al. AHA/ACCF Secondary Preven-tion and Risk Reduction Therapy for Patients with Coronary and Other Atherosclerotic Vascular Disease: 2011 Update. A Guideline from the American Heart Association and American College of Cardiology Foun-dation. Circulation 2011; 124:00–000.

Roger VL, Go AS, Lloyd-Jones DM, et al. Heart disease and stroke statis-tics--2011 update: a report from the American Heart Association. Circu-lation 2011;123:e18-e209.

Weintraub WS, Daniels SR, Burke LE, et al. Value of Primordial and Pri-mary Prevention for Cardiovascular Disease: A Policy Statement From the American Heart Association. Circulation. Aug 23 2011; 124(8): 967-990.

Ebrahim S, Taylor F, Ward K, Beswick A, Burke M, Davey Smith G. Multiple risk factor interventions for primary prevention of coronary heart disease. Cochrane Database Syst Rev. Jan 19 2011; CD001561.

National Heart, Lung, and Blood Institute (NHLBI). Estimate of 10-Year Risk for Coronary Heart Disease Framingham Point Scores. Available at http://www.nhlbi.nih.gov/guidelines/cholesterol/risk_tbl.htm.

Greenland P, Alpert JS, Beller GA, et al. 2010 ACCF/AHA guideline for assessment of cardiovascular risk in asymptomatic adults: executive summary: a report of the American College of Cardiology Foundation/American Heart Association Task Force on Practice Guidelines. J Am Coll Cardiol. Dec 14 2010; 56(25):2182-99.

MRC/BHF Heart Protection Study of cholesterol lowering with simvastatin in 20,536 high-risk individuals: a randomised placebo-controlled trial. Lancet. Jul 6 2002; 360(9326):7-22.

Balagopal PB, de Ferranti SD, Cook S, et al. Nontraditional Risk Factors and Biomarkers for Cardiovascular Disease: Mechanistic, Research, and Clinical Considerations for Youth: A Scientific Statement From the American Heart Association. Circulation. Jun 14 2011; 123(23): 2749–2769.

Rozanski A, Gransar H, Shaw LJ, et al. Impact of Coronary Artery Calcium Scanning on Coronary Risk Factors and Downstream Testing The EISNER (Early Identification of Subclinical Atherosclerosis by Noninvasive Imaging Research) Prospective Randomized Trial. J Am Coll Cardiol. Apr 12 2011; 57(15):1622–32.

Yusuf S, Lonn E, Bosch J. Lipid lowering for primary prevention. Lancet. Apr 4 2009; 373(9670):1152–5.

Teo KK, Ounpuu S, Hawken S, Pandey MR, Valentin V, Hunt D, et al. Tobacco use and risk of myocardial infarction in 52 countries in the INTERHEART study: a case-control study. Lancet. Aug 19 2006; 368 (9536):647–58.

Wang TD, Chen WJ, Chien KL, Seh-Yi Su SS, Hsu HC, Chen MF, et al. Efficacy of cholesterol levels and ratios in predicting future coronary heart disease in a Chinese population. Am J Cardiol. Oct 1 2001; 88(7):737–43.

National Heart, Lung, and Blood Institute (NHLBI). ATP III Update 2004: Implications of Recent Clinical Trials for the ATP III Guidelines. NIH.

Available at http://www.nhlbi.nih.gov/guidelines/cholesterol/atp3upd04. pdf.

Bulbulia R, Bowman L, Wallendszus K, Parish S, Armitage J, Peto R, et al. Effects on 11-year mortality and morbidity of lowering LDL cholesterol with simvastatin for about 5 years in 20,536 high-risk individuals: a randomised controlled trial. Lancet. Dec 10 2011; 378(9808): 2013–20.

Blaha MJ, Budoff MJ, DeFilippis AP, et al. Associations between C-reactive protein, coronary artery calcium, and cardiovascular events: implications for the JUPITER population from MESA, a population-based cohort study. Lancet. Aug 20 2011;378(9792):684-92.

Lipids and lipoproteins in symptomatic coronary heart disease. Distribution, intercorrelations, and significance for risk classification in 6,700 men and 1,500 women. The Bezafibrate Infarction Prevention (BIP) Study Group, Israel. Circulation. Sep 1992; 86(3):839–48.

Third Report of the National Cholesterol Education Program (NCEP) Expert Panel on Detection, Evaluation, and Treatment of High Blood Cholesterol in Adults (Adult Treatment Panel III) final report. Circulation. Dec 17 2002;106(25):3143–421.

Le NA, Walter MF. The role of hypertriglyceridemia in atherosclerosis. Curr Atheroscler Rep. Aug 2007; 9(2):110–5.

Yuan G, Al-Shali KZ, Hegele RA. Hypertriglyceridemia: its etiology, effects and treatment. CMAJ. Apr 10 2007;176(8):1113-20.

Frick MH, Elo O, Haapa K, Heinonen OP, Heinsalmi P, Helo P, et al. Helsinki Heart Study: primary-prevention trial with gemfibrozil in middle-aged men with dyslipidemia. Safety of treatment, changes in risk factors, and incidence of coronary heart disease. N Engl J Med. Nov 12 1987; 317(20):1237–45.

McManus RJ, Mant J, Bray EP, Holder R, Jones MI, Greenfield S. Telemonitoring and self-management in the control of hypertension (TASMINH2): a randomised controlled trial. Lancet. Jul 17 2010; 376(9736): 163–72.

Jenkins DJ, Kendall CW, Marchie A, Faulkner DA, Wong JM, de Souza R, et al. Effects of a dietary portfolio of cholesterol-lowering foods vs. lovastatin on serum lipids and C-reactive protein. JAMA. Jul 23 2003; 290(4): 502-10.

Kastorini CM, Milionis HJ, Esposito K, Giugliano D, Goudevenos JA, Panagiotakos DB. The effect of mediterranean diet on metabolic syndrome and its components a meta-analysis of 50 studies and 534,906 individuals. J Am Coll Cardiol. Mar 15 2011; 57(11):1299–313.

Nordmann AJ, Suter-Zimmermann K, Bucher HC, et al. Meta-analysis comparing mediterranean to low-fat diets for modification of cardiovascular risk factors. Am J Med. Sep 2011;124(9):841–851.e2.

Yusuf S, Dagenais G, Pogue J, Bosch J, Sleight P. Vitamin E supplementation and cardiovascular events in high-risk patients. The Heart Outcomes Prevention Evaluation Study Investigators. N Engl J Med. Jan 20 2000; 342(3):154–60.

Asplund K. Antioxidant vitamins in the prevention of cardiovascular disease: a systematic review. J Intern Med. May 2002;251(5):372–92.

SMOKING CESSATION

Hermanson B, Omenn GS, Kronmal RA, Gersh BJ. Beneficial six-year outcome of smoking cessation in older men and women with coronary artery disease. Results from the CASS registry. N Engl J Med. Nov 24 1988; 319(21):1365–9.

Critchley JA, Capewell S. Mortality risk reduction associated with smoking cessation in patients with coronary heart disease: a systematic review. JAMA. Jul 2 2003;290(1):86–97.

Pearson TA, Blair SN, Daniels SR, Eckel RH, Fair JM, Fortmann SP. AHA Guidelines for Primary Prevention of Cardiovascular Disease and Stroke: 2002 Update: Consensus Panel Guide to Comprehensive Risk Reduction for Adult Patients Without Coronary or Other Atherosclerotic Vascular Diseases. American Heart Association Science Advisory and Coordinating Committee. Circulation. Jul 16 2002; 106(3):388-91.

Berger JS, Lala A, Krantz MJ, Baker GS, Hiatt WR. Aspirin for the prevention of cardiovascular events in patients without clinical cardiovascular disease: A meta-analysis of randomized trials. Am Heart J. Jul 2011; 162(1):115-124.e2.

Smith SC Jr, Allen J, Blair SN, Bonow RO, Brass LM, Fonarow GC, et al. AHA/ACC guidelines for secondary prevention for patients with coronary and other atherosclerotic vascular disease: 2006 update: endorsed by the National Heart, Lung, and Blood Institute. Circulation. May 16 2006; 113(19):2363-72.

Greenland P, Alpert JS, Beller GA, et al. 2010 ACCF/AHA guideline for assessment of cardiovascular risk in asymptomatic adults: a report of the

American College of Cardiology Foundation/American Heart Association Task Force on Practice Guidelines. Circulation. Dec 21 2010; 122(25): e584-636.

Sattelmair J, Pertman J, Ding EL, et al. Dose response between physical activity and risk of coronary heart disease: a meta-analysis. Circulation. Aug 16 2011; 124(7):789-95.

Mosca L, Appel LJ, Benjamin EJ, Berra K, Chandra-Strobos N, Fabunmi RP, et al. Evidence-based guidelines for cardiovascular disease prevention in women. Circulation. Feb 10 2004;109(5):672-93.

Ascherio A. Hennekens CH, Buring JE, et al. Trans-fatty acids intake and risk of myocardial infarction. Circulation. Jan 1994; 89(1):94-101.

Chobanian AV, Bakris GL, Black HR, et al. The Seventh Report of the Joint National Committee on Prevention, Detection, Evaluation, and Treatment of High Blood Pressure: the JNC 7 report. JAMA. 289(19): 2560-72.

Executive Summary of The Third Report of The National Cholesterol Education Program (NCEP) Expert Panel on Detection, Evaluation, and Treatment of High Blood Cholesterol In Adults (Adult Treatment Panel III). JAMA. May 16 2001; 285(19):2486–97.

Hakim AA, Curb JD, Petrovitch H, et al. Effects of walking on coronary heart disease in elderly men: the Honolulu Heart Program. Circulation. Jul 6 1999;100(1):9–13.

DINE FOR 5 EAT FOR 1: DIETS FOR HEART DISEASE

Hu FB, Willett WC. Optimal diets for prevention of coronary heart disease. JAMA. Nov 27 2002; 288(20):2569–78.

Jha P, Flather M, Lonn E, et al. The antioxidant vitamins and cardiovascular disease. A critical review of epidemiologic and clinical trial data. Ann Intern Med. Dec 1 1995;123(11):860-72.

Key TJ, Thorogood M, Appleby PN, Burr ML. Dietary habits and mortality in 11,000 vegetarians and health conscious people: results of a 17 year follow up. BMJ. Sep 28 1996;313(7060):775–9.

Law MR, Morris JK. By how much does fruit and vegetable consumption reduce the risk of ischaemic heart disease?. Eur J Clin Nutr. Aug 1998; 52(8):549–56.

Manson JE, Hu FB, Rich-Edwards JW, et al. A prospective study of walking as compared with vigorous exercise in the prevention of coronary heart disease in women. N Engl J Med. Aug 26 1999; 341(9):650–8.

Pietinen P, Rimm EB, Korhonen P, et al. Intake of dietary fiber and risk of coronary heart disease in a cohort of Finnish men. The Alpha-Tocopherol, Beta-Carotene Cancer Prevention Study. Circulation. Dec 1 1996; 94(11):2720–7.

Rimm EB. Alcohol consumption and coronary heart disease: good habits may be more important than just good wine. Am J Epidemiol. Jun 1 1996; 143(11):1094-8; discussion 1099.

Rimm EB, Ascherio A, Giovannucci E, et al. Vegetable, fruit, and cereal fiber intake and risk of coronary heart disease among men. JAMA. Feb 14 1996; 275(6):447–51.

Chomistek A, Cook N, Flint A, Rimm E. Vigorous-intensity leisure-time physical activity and risk of major chronic disease in men. Med Sci Sports Exerc. April 24 2012.

NOTES

CHAPTER 1

1. Topol, Eric J., "Randomised placebo-controlled and balloon-angio-plasty-controlled trial to assess safety of coronary stenting with use of plate-let glycoprotein-IIb/IIIa blockade," *The Lancet*, 9122 (2009): 87–92. Accessed September 4, 2013, doi:10.1016/S0140-6736(98)85010-1.

2. Roger VL, Go AS, Lloyd-Jones DM, Benjamin EJ, Berry JD, Borden WB, et al. "Heart disease and stroke statistics—2012 update: a report from the American Heart Association," *Circulation*, 125 (2012): pp 2–220. Accessed September 6, 2013, doi: 10.1161/ CIR.0b013e31823ac046.

3. Bowden, WE, et al, "Optimal medical therapy with or without PCI for stable coronary disease," *New England Journal of Medicine*, 356, (2007) 15:1503–16. Accessed September 6, 2013, http://www.nejm.org/doi/full /10.1056/NEJMoa070829.

4. Miglioretti, DL, et al, "The use of computed tomography in pediatrics and the associated radiation exposure and estimated cancer risks," *JAMA Pediatrics*. 2013 Aug 1; 167(8): 700–7. doi: 10.1001/jamapediatrics.2013 .311.

5. Pascal Meier, et al, "The impact of the coronary collateral circulation on mortality: a meta-analysis," *European Heart Journal*, 33 (2012) 5: 614–621. Accessed September 12, 2013, doi:10.1093/eurheartj/ehr308.

6. Heidenreich, Paul A, et al, "Forecasting the Future of Cardiovascular Disease in the United States: A Policy Statement From the American Heart

Association," *Circulation,* 123 (2011) 123: 933–944. Accessed September 4, 2013, doi:10.1161/CIR.0b013e31820a55f5.

7. "Heart Disease May Be on the Rise Again, After Years of Decline, Population Research Shows," Science Daily. Accessed September 12, 2013, http://www.sciencedaily.com /releases/2008/02/080211172623.htm.

8. "AHA Statistical Update: Heart Disease and Stroke Statistics—2013 Update," *Circulation,*127 (2013): 6–245. Accessed September 11, 2013, doi: 10.1161/ CIR.0b013e31828124ad.

9. "Obesity and Overweight," Centers for Disease Control and Prevention, last modified 2010, http://www.cdc.gov/nchs/fastats/overwt.htm.

10. Rena R. Phelan, Suzanne Wing, "Long Term Weight Loss Maintenance," *American Journal of Clinical Nutrition,* 82 (2005): 2225–2255. Accessed September 6, 2013, http://ajcn.nutrition.org/content/82/1/222S.full.

CHAPTER 2

1. Mark Hyman, MD, "8 Steps to Reversing Diabesity," Dr. Mark Hyman, May 4, 2013, accessed September 6, 2013, http://drhyman.com/blog/2011/11/17/8-steps-to-reversing-diabesity/.

2. "Computed Tomography to Detect Coronary Artery Calcification," *Cigna Healthcare Coverage Position,* (2006): 1–14. Accessed October 21, 2013, https://my.cigna.com/teamsite/health/provider/medical/procedural/coverage_positions/medical/mm_0009_coveragepositioncriteria_electron_beam_ct_for_cad.pdf.

3. "Heart Disease Facts and Statistics," CDC, modified October 16, 2012, accessed September 6, 2013, http://www.cdc.gov/heartdisease/statistics .htm.

4. "Lifestyle Medicine Strategies for Risk Factor Reduction, Prevention, and Treatment of Coronary Heart Disease: Part II," American Journal of Lifestyle Medicine, accessed September 3, 2013, http://ajl.sagepub.com/content/1/2/79.abstract.

5. Eric A. Finkelstein, et al, "Obesity and Severe Obesity Forecasts Through 2030," *American Journal of Preventive Medicine,* 42 (2012) 6: 563–570. Accessed September 9, 2013, http://www.ajpmonline.org/article/S0749-3797(12)00146-8/abstract.

6. Liping Pan, et al, "Incidences of obesity and extreme obesity among US adults: findings from the 2009 Behavioral Risk Factor Surveillance

System," *Population Health Metrics*, 56(2011), accessed September 6, 2013, doi:10.1186/1478-7954-9-56.

7. Bruce Neal, "Fat chance for physical activity," *Population Health Metrics,* July 10 2013, accessed September 6, 2013, 11:9 doi:10.1186/1478 -7954-11-9.

8. Michael Specter, *Denialism: How Irrational Thinking Hinders Scientific Progress, Harms the Planet, and Threatens Our Lives,* (New York: The Penguin Press, 2009), kindle edition.

9. Laurian Unnevehr, "Crop Case Study: GMO Golden Rice in Asia with Enhanced Vitamin A Benefits for Consumers," *AgBioFourm,* 10 (2007): 154-60. Accessed September 6, 2013, http://www.agbioforum.org/v10n3/v10n3a04-unnevehr.htm.

CHAPTER 3

1. "Metabolic Syndrome Explained by its Discoverer," Insulite Laboratories, accessed September 3, 2013, http://metabolic-syndrome.insu-litelabs.com/Metabolic-Syndrome-Explained.php.

2. "High-Intensity Intermittent Exercise and Fat Loss," *Journal of Obesity*, accessed September 4, 2013, http://www.ncbi.nlm.nih.gov/pmc/articles/PMC2991639/.

3. "Skeletal Muscle Insulin Resistance Promotes Increased Hepatic De Novo Lipogenesis, Hyperlipidemia, and Hepatic Steatosis in the Elderly," Diabetes, accessed September 3, 2013, http://diabetes.diabetesjournals.org/content/61/11/2711.full; "Metabolic Syndrome: Don't Blame the Belly Fat," HHMI News, accessed September 3, 2013, http://www.hhmi.org/news/metabolic-syndrome-dont-blame-belly-fat.

4. "High Blood Pressure Facts," Centers for Disease Control and Prevention, accessed September 6, 2013, http://www.cdc.gov/bloodpres-sure/facts.htm.

5. "AHA Scientific Statement: Triglycerides and Cardiovascular Disease," Circulation, accessed September 3, 2013, http://circ.ahajournals.org/con-tent/123/20/2292.long.

6. "Race/Ethnic Disparities in Utilization of Lifesaving Technologies by Medicare Ischemic Heart Disease Beneficiaries," Medical Care, accessed September 3, 2013, http://journals.lww.com/lww-medicalcare/Abstract/2005/04000/Race_Ethnic_Disparities_in_Utilization_of.4.aspx.

7. "Obesity and African Americans," U.S. Department of Health and Human Services, September 6, 2013, http://minorityhealth.hhs.gov/templates/content.aspx?ID=6456.

8. "Overweight and Obesity Statistics," U.S. Department of Health and Human Services, accessed September 6, 2013, http://win.niddk.nih.gov/publications/PDFs/stat904z.pdf.

CHAPTER 4

1. "Vital Signs: Awareness and Treatment of Uncontrolled Hypertension Among Adults — United States, 2003–2010," *Centers for Disease Control and Prevention*, 61 (2012) 35: 703-709. Accessed September 9, 2013, http://www.cdc.gov/mmwr/preview/mmwrhtml/mm6135a3.htmhttp://www.cdc.gov/mmwr/preview/mmwrhtml/mm6135a3.htm?s_cid=mm6135a3_w.

2. "What Is High Blood Pressure," *National Heart, Lung and Blood Institute* (NHLBI), accessed September 9, 2013, http://www.nhlbi.nih.gov/health/health-topics/topics/hbp/.

3. Ibid.

CHAPTER 5

1. "National Prevention, Health Promotion, and Public Health Council," http://www.surgeongeneral.gov/initiatives/prevention/strategy/report.pdf

2. "Exercise nearly as successful as drugs at lowering blood sugar," University of Michigan New Service, accessed September 4, 2013, http://www.ur.umich.edu/0506/Nov21_05/06.shtml.

3. Francisco B. Ortega, et al, "The intriguing metabolically healthy but obese phenotype: cardiovascular prognosis and role of fitness," *European Heart Journal*, 34 (2013) 5: 389-397. Accessed September 10, 2013, doi:10.1093/eurheartj/ehs174.

4. "Exercise's Effect on the Heart," reprinted in the *New York Times*, accessed September 4, 2013, http://health.nytimes.com/health/guides/specialtopic/physical-activity/exercise's-effects-on-the-heart.html.

CHAPTER 6

1. Van Dis I, Kromhout D, Geleijnse M, et al., "Body mass index and waist circumference predict both 10-year non-fatal and fatal cardiovascular

disease risk in 20,000 Dutch men and women aged 20-65," *Eur J Cardiovasc Prev Rehabil*, 2009; DOI: 10.1097/HJR.0b013e328331dfc0.

2. CJ Lavie, et al, "Obesity and cardiovascular disease: risk factor, paradox, and impact of weight loss," *Journal of the American College of Cardiology*, 26 (2009): 1925–32. doi: 10.1016/j.jacc.2008.12.068.

3. "Combining Body Mass Index With Measures of Central Obesity in the Assessment of Mortality in Subjects With Coronary Disease," Journal of the American College of Cardiology, accessed September 4, 2013, http://content.onlinejacc.org/article.aspx?articleid=1559955.

4. Ishwarial Jialal, "Increased Chemerin and Decreased Omentin-1 in Both Adipose Tissue and Plasma in Nascent Metabolic Syndrome," *The Journal of Clinical Endocrinology & Metabolism*, 9 (2013): 2012–3673. Accessed September 8, 2013, doi: 10.1210/jc.2012-3673.

CHAPTER 7

1. "National Diabetes Statistics 2011," The U.S. Department of Health and Human Services.

2. Erika Gebel, "The Other Diabetes: LADA, or Type 5," *Diabetes Forecast*, May 2010, accessed October 22, 2013, http://forecast.diabetes.org/magazine/features/other-diabetes-lada-or-type-15.

3. Barbara B. Kahn and Jeffrey S. Flier, "Obesity and insulin resistance," *The Journal of Clinical Investigation*, 106 (2000) 4:473–481. Accessed September 12, 2013, doi:10.1172/JCI10842.

4. Crane, Paul K, et al, "Glucose Levels and Risk of Dementia," *New England Journal of Medicine*, (2013); 369: 540-48, accessed October 21, 2013, DOI: 10.1056/NEJMoa1215740.

5. Richard S. Surwit, Mark S. Schneider, and Mark N. Feinglos, "Stress and Diabetes Mellitus," *Diabetes Care*, 15 (1992) 10: 1413-1422. Accessed September 9, 2013, doi: 10.2337/diacare.15.10.1413.

CHAPTER 8

1. "Saturated Fats vs. unsaturated fats," Diff/en, accessed September 4, 2013, http://www.diffen.com/difference/Saturated_Fats_vs_Unsaturated_Fats.

2. Beatrice Alexandra Golomb, Michael H. Criqui, Halbert White, Joel E. Dimsdale, "Conceptual Foundations of the UCSD Statin Study: A

Randomized Controlled Trial Assessing the Impact of Statins on Cognition, Behavior, and Biochemistry," *JAMA Internal Medicine,* 164(2004)2: 153–162. Accessed September 13, 2013, doi:10.1001/archinte.164.2.153.

3. Chittaranjan Andrade and Rajiv Radhakrishnan, "The prevention and treatment of cognitive decline and dementia: An overview of recent research on experimental treatments," *Indian Journal of Psychiatry,* 51 (2009) 1: 12–25. Accessed September 9, 2013, http://www.ncbi.nlm.nih.gov/pmc/articles/PMC2738400/.

4. Mason W. Freeman, M.D. with Christine Junge, "Understanding Cholesterol: The Good, the Bad, and the Necessary" in *The Harvard Medical School Guide to Lowering Your Cholesterol* (New York: The McGraw Hill Companies, 2005), Chapter 1.

5. Campbell, T. Colin, PhD, with Thomas M. Campbell II, *The China Study: Startling Implications for Diet, Weight Loss, and Long-Term Health,* Dallas: BenBella Books, 2004, p. 151.

6. Gustavo Bounous, Francine Gervais, Victor Amer, Gerald Batist, and Phil Gold, "The Influence of Dietary Whey Protein on Tissue Glutathione and the Diseases Of Aging," *Journal of Clinical and Investigative Medicine,* 12 (1989) 6: 343–9. Accessed September 12, 2013, http://www.ncbi.nlm.nih.gov/pubmed/2692897.

7. P. Micke, K. M. Beeh, J. F. Schlaak, R. Buhl, "Oral supplementation with whey proteins increases plasma glutathione levels of HIV-infected patients," *European Journal of Clinical Investigation,* 31 (2001) 2: 171–8. Accessed September 12, 2013, DOI: 10.1046/j.1365-2362.2001.00781.x.

8. "Associations Between Acute Lipid Stress Responses and Fasting Lipid Levels 3 Years Later," *Health Psychology,* accessed September 4, 2013, http://www.apa.org/pubs/journals/releases/hea-246601.pdf.

9. David Perlmutter, M.D., *Grain Brain* (New York: Little, Brown and Company, 2013).

CHAPTER 9

1. Dwyer, Joanna T., Ouyang, Chung Mei, "What can industry do to facilitate dietary and behavioural changes," *British Journal of Nutrition,* 83 (2000): S173-S180. Accessed September 5, 2013, DOI: http://dx.doi.org/10.1017/S0007114500001136. University Of North Carolina at Chapel Hill (2003, January 22). UNC Study Confirms That Food Portion Sizes Increased in U.S. Over Two Decades. *ScienceDaily.* Retrieved

September 5, 2013, from http://www.sciencedaily.com /releases/2003/01/ 030122072329.htm.

2. Sumithran, Priya, et al. "Long-Term Persistence of Hormonal Adaptations to Weight Loss," *N Engl J Med* 2011; 365:1597–1604 October 27, 2011DOI: 10.1056/NEJMoa1105816.

3. "Dieting Does Not Work," UCLA Researchers Report, accessed September 5 2013, http://newsroom.ucla.edu/portal/ucla/dieting-does-not-work-ucla-researchers-7832.aspx.

4. "Adult Obesity Facts," Centers for Disease Control and Prevention, accessed September 5, 2013, http://www.cdc.gov/obesity/data/adult.html.

5. Narayan KMV, Boyle JP, Geiss LS, Saaddine JB, Thompson TJ. "Impact of Recent Increase in Incidence on Future Diabetes Burden U.S., 2005–2050," *Diabetes Care,* 29 (2006): 2114-2116. Accessed September 5, 2013, doi: 10.2337/dc06-1136.

6. Behan, Donald F., et al, "Obesity and its Relation to Mortality and Morbidity Costs," *Society of Actuaries,* 2010: 1–80.

7. Casazza, Kristen, et al, "Myths, Presumptions, and Facts about Obesity," *N Engl J Med* 2013; 368:446-454. Accessed September 5 2013, DOI: 10.1056/NEJMsa1208051.

8. "Childhood Obesity," Children's Defense Fund, accessed September 5, 2013, http://www.childrensdefense.org/policy-priorities/childrens-health/child-nutrition/childhood-obesity.html.

9. Wilen, John, "Gas stations look in store for profits," *USA Today* online, accessed September 5, 2013, http://usatoday30.usatoday.com/money/economy/2008-04-01-4185633325_x.htm.

10. Gretchen Voss, "Weight Loss Help: How to Lose Weight and Keep It Off," *Women's Health Online,* April 13, 2012.

11. "Portion Distortion and Serving Size," National Heart, Lung and Blood Institute, accessed September 9, 2013, http://www.nhlbi.nih.gov/health/public/heart/obesity/wecan/eat-right/distortion.htm.

12. Lisa R. Young, Marion Nestle, "Portion Sizes and Obesity: Responses of Fast-Food Companies," *Journal of Public Health Policy,* 28 (July 2007), 238–248. Accessed September 8, 2013, doi:10.1057/palgrave.jphp. 3200127.

13. Jane Ogden, "Distraction, the desire to eat and food intake. Towards an expanded model of mindless eating," *Appetite,* 62 (2013) 1: 119026. Accessed September 9, 2013, http://dx.doi.org/10.1016/j.appet.2012.11 .023.

14. Brian Wansink, Koert van Ittersum, James E. Painter "Ice Cream Illusions: Bowls, Spoons, and Self-Served Portion Sizes," *American Journal of Preventive Medicine* 31 (2006) 3: 240–243, accessed September 8, 2013, DOI: 10.1016/j.amepre.2006.04.003.

15. Nicole M. Avena, Pedro Rada, Bartley G. Hoebel, "Evidence for sugar addiction: Behavioral and neurochemical effects of intermittent, excessive sugar intake," *Neuroscience and Biobehavioral Reviews,* 32 (2008) 1: 20–39. Accessed September 8, 2013, http://www.ncbi.nlm.nih.gov/pubmed/17617461.

16. National Weight Control Registry. Accessed September 8, 2013.

17. Mashid Dehghan, et al, "Relationship Between Healthy Diet and Risk of Cardiovascular Disease Among Patients on Drug Therapies for Secondary Prevention," *Circulation,* 126 (2012): 2705–2712. Accessed September 8, 2013, doi: 10.1161/ CIRCULATIONAHA.112.103234.

CHAPTER 10

1. "Fast Facts, The Centers for Disease Control and Prevention," accessed September 6, 2013, http://www.cdc.gov/tobacco/data_statistics/fact_sheets/fast_facts/.

2. "Childhood Obesity Facts," CDC, accessed September 6, 2013, http://www.cdc.gov/healthyyouth/obesity/facts.htm.

3. "Obesity in Children and Teens," *Amercan Academy of Child & Adolescent Psychiatry,* 79 (2011), accessed September 6, 2013, http://www.aacap.org/AACAP/Families_and_Youth/Facts_for_Families/Facts_for_Families_Pages/Obesity_In_Children_And_Teens_79.aspx.

4. Hadfield, SC, Preece, PM, "Obesity in looked after children: is foster care protective from the dangers of obesity," *Child Care Health Dev,* 2008 Nov; 34(6):710-2. doi: 10.1111/j.1365-2214.2008.00874.x.

5. Hamrick, Karen S., et al, "How Much Time Do Americans Spend on Food," USDA Economic Research Service, 86 (2011), accessed September 6, 2013, http://www.ers.usda.gov/media/149404/eib86.pdf.

6. Michael Pollan, *Cooked: A Natural History of Transformation* (New York: Penguin Press HC, 2013), 88–90.

7. Reis, Jared P, et al, "Association Between Duration of Overall and Abdominal Obesity Beginning in Young Adulthood and Coronary Artery Calcification in Middle Age," *JAMA,* 2013; 310(3):280–288. doi:10.1001/jama.2013.7833.

8. De Ferranti, Sarah, "NHLBI guidelines on cholesterol in kids: What's new and how does this change practice," *AAP NEWS*, Vol. 33 No. 2 February 1, 2012: 1. Accessed September 6, 2013, doi: 10.1542/aapnews. 2012332-1b).

9. "A Review of Food Marketing to Children and Adolescents," *Federal Trade Commission Report, 2012:* pp 61–90. Accessed September 6, 2013, http://www.ftc.gov/os/2012/12/121221foodmarketingreport.pdf.

10. Cara Wilking, "Issue Brief: Reining in Pester Power Food and Beverage Marketing," *The Public Health Advocacy Institute,* pp. 1–9. Accessed September 6, 2013, http://www.phaionline.org/wp-content/uploads/2011/09/Pester_power.pdf.

11. Jennifer L. Harris, et al, "Food marketing to children and adolescents: What do parents think," *Rudd Report,* 2012, pp. 1–48. Accessed September 6, 2013, http://www.yaleruddcenter.org/resources/upload/docs/what/reports/Rudd_Report_Parents_Survey_Food_Marketing_2012.pdf.

12. "Current Tobacco Use Among Middle and High School Students – United States, 2011," *Centers for Disease Control and Prevention (CDC). MMWR.* 2012;61(31):581-585. Accessed September 6, 2013, at www.cdc.gov/mmwr/preview/mmwrhtml/mm6131a1.htm?s_cid=mm6131a1_w#tab.

13. "Smoking and Tabacco Use," *Centers for Disease Control and Prevention Fact Sheet,* accessed September 6, 2013, http://www.cdc.gov/tobacco/data_statistics/fact_sheets/fast_facts/.

CHAPTER 11

1. Daniel Ariely, *Predicatbly Irrational: The Hidden Forces That Shape Our Decisions* (New York: Harper Perrenial 2010), Kindle edition.

INDEX